C000179461

PROSTATIC OUTFLOW OBSTRUCTION: CLINICAL INVESTIGATION AND TREATMENT

Prostatic Outflow Obstruction: Clinical Investigation and Treatment

EDITED BY

P.J.R. SHAH FRCS

Senior Lecturer, Institute of Urology
Consultant Urologist to St Peter's Hospital
at the Middlesex Hospital, London
and to the Royal National Orthopaedic
Hospital Trust, Stanmore

FOREWORD BY

J.E.A. WICKHAM

MS BSc FRCS FRCP FRCR
Consultant Urologist
29 Devonshire Place
London

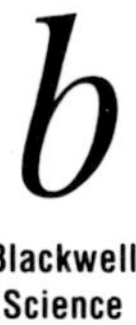

Blackwell
Science

Editorial Offices:
Osney Mead, Oxford OX2 0EL
25 John Street, London WC1N 2BL
23 Ainslie Place, Edinburgh EH3 6AJ
238 Main Street, Cambridge
Massachusetts 02142, USA
54 University Street, Carlton
Victoria 3053, Australia

Other Editorial Offices:
Arnette Blackwell SA
1, rue de Lille
75007 Paris
France

Blackwell Wissenschafts-Verlag GmbH
Düsseldorfer Str. 38
D-10707 Berlin
Germany

Blackwell MZV
Feldgasse 13
A-1238 Wien
Austria

First published 1994

Set by Setrite Typesetters, Hong Kong
Printed and bound in Great Britain
at the University Press, Cambridge

DISTRIBUTORS

Marston Book Services Ltd
PO Box 87
Oxford OX2 0DT
(*Orders*: Tel: 01865 791155
Fax: 01865 791927
Telex: 837515)

North America
Blackwell Science, Inc.
238 Main Street
Cambridge, MA 02142
(*Orders*: Tel: 800 215–1000
617 876–7000
Fax: 617 492–5263)

Australia
Blackwell Science Pty Ltd
54 University Street
Carlton, Victoria 3053
(*Orders*: Tel: 03 347-5552)

A catalogue record for this title is available from the British Library

ISBN 0-632-03557-9

Library of Congress
Cataloging-in-Publication Data

Prostatic outflow obstruction: clinical investigation and treatment/
edited by P.J.R. Shah.
p. cm.
Includes bibliographical references and index.
ISBN 0-632-03557-9
1. Prostate — Diseases. I. Shah, P.J.R.
[DNLM: 1. Prostatic Diseases — therapy.
2. Prostatic Diseases — diagnosis. WJ 752
A244 1994]
RC899.A33 1994
616.6′5 — dc20

Contents

List of Contributors

D.G. BARNES MB ChB FRCS
Senior Registrar in Urology, Leicester General Hospital, Gwendolen Road, Leicester, LE5 4PW

B.R.P. BIRCH MA FRCS
Senior Registrar in Urology, Southampton University Hospital, Tremona Road, Southampton, SO9 4XY

C.R. CHARIG MB BS MA FRCS (Urol)
Consultant Urologist, Epsom General Hospital, Dorking Road, Epsom, Surrey, KT18 7EG

S.W.V. COPPINGER MB FRCS FRCSE
Senior Registrar in Urology, St Peter's Hospital, Henrietta Street, London, WC2

G. DAS MS FRCS (Urol)
Consultant Urologist, Mayday University Hospital, Thornton Heath, Surrey, CR7 7YE

C. HUDD MS FRCS (Urol) FEBU
Senior Registrar in Urology, Wexham Park Hospital, Slough, Berkshire, SL2 4HC

P.F. KEANE MCH FRCS (Urol)
Consultant Urologist, Level 3, City Hospital, Lisburn Road, Belfast, BT9 7AB

R.A. MILLER MS FRCS
Consultant and Post-Graduate Dean, Whittington and Royal Northern Hospitals, Department of Urology, St Mary's Wing, Highgate Hill, London, N19 5NF

E.J. MILROY MB BS FRCS LRCP
Consultant Urologist, Middlesex Hospital, Mortimer Street, London, W1N 8AA

T. McNICHOLAS MB BS FRCS
Department of Urology, Lister Hospital, N. Herts Trust, Corey's Mill Lane, Stevenage, Herts, SG1 4AB

B.C. OGBONA
Urology Unit, Department of Surgery, Jos University Teaching Hospital, PME 2076, Jos, Nigeria

A.P. PERLMUTTER
Director of Prostate Unit, Cornell University Hospital, New York, USA

List of Contributors

P.J.R. SHAH FRCS
Senior Lecturer, Institute of Urology, Consultant Urologist to St Peter's Hospital at the Middlesex Hospital, London and to the Royal National Orthopaedic Hospital Trust, Stanmore

T.K. SHAH MB BS LRCP FRCS
Department of Urology, Lister Hospital, N. Herts Trust, Corey's Mill Lane, Stevenage, Herts, SG1 4AB

G.M. WATSON MD BChir MB FRCS
Whittington and Royal Northern Hospitals, Department of Urology, St Mary's Wing, Highgate Hill, London, N19 5NF

J.E.A. WICKHAM MS BSc FRCS FRCP FRCR
Consultant Urologist, 29 Devonshire Place, London, W1N 1PE

Foreword

'A flayed mouse dried and beaten into a powder helps such as cannot hold their water.' (Nicholas Culpepper, 1600)

In reviewing the many new treatments recommended for prostatism over the last 10 years it would sometimes appear that if this seventeenth-century remedy were to be presented currently as a scientific paper, there would be some who would proclaim its therapeutic efficacy with enthusiasm! The multiplicity of new methods described and acclaimed since 1980 has been quite extraordinary, and to gain some objective sense of the situation the members of the Academic Unit of the Institute of Urology in London have undertaken a comprehensive review and evaluation of the various new therapies being advocated.

This volume is the result of their efforts, and it examines the currently described techniques for the relief of prostatism.

The problem of benign prostatic obstruction seems a simple one in hydrostatic terms: a flow tube is circumferentially obstructed mainly by glandular tissue with a relatively high proportion of hard white fibrous tissue stroma. The primary solution is therefore one of bulk removal, very well achieved previously by open prostatic adenectomy and subsequently by piecemeal removal by transurethral resection. The result of these techniques has generally been very satisfactory, but at the cost of some patient discomfort and inconvenience. The desire of clinicians to obviate these perioperative problems has led to the investigation of alternative methods that will be able to achieve diminution of prostatic bulk without associated morbidity.

The new therapies must therefore be measured against the yardstick of how well they achieve reduction in adenoma size versus the complications induced by the method. A thorough understanding of the anatomy of the region and of methods of assessment of the clinical problem is essential to this aim, and has been addressed in Chapters 1 and 2. The truly non-invasive medical management is reviewed in Chapter 3, and ultrasound-guided techniques in Chapter 4. Chapter 5 contains a discussion of balloon dilatation of benign prostatic hypertrophy. Prostatic hyperthermia is comprehensively reviewed in Chapter 6 and prostatic stenting in Chapter 9. Chapters 7 and 8 deal with the mysterious disease of chronic prostatitis. Transurethral resection of the prostate under local anaesthesia, blood loss in transurethral surgery and the use of lasers in benign prostatic hypertrophy and in the malignant prostate are examined in Chapters 10, 11 and 12 respectively.

I think for the forseeable future transurethral diathermy resection will be the mainstay of the armamentarium. It is effective and has stood the test of time over many years. For the reasons given in the text I believe laser therapy will establish a firm place for itself when some of its limitations have been overcome. Techniques which are currently being evaluated such as robotic prostatectomy and extra-corporeal ultrasound tissue ablation may well come to occupy a more important position in the treatment spectrum in time.

Whatever method is adopted however, bulk removal of tissue would seem to be the prime requisite of success. If this can be achieved elegantly with low morbidity and zero mortality then our patients will be truly served. This book provides a concise guide to this important subject.

J. E. A. Wickham

Preface

During the late 1980s, the Institute of Urology under the Directorship of Mr J.E.A. Wickham had embarked upon a variety of research projects into the treatment of prostatic outflow obstruction. Some of these investigations and treatment methods were in general clinical use and some were innovations directed by minimally invasive approaches to management.

As a consequence of the large number of projects during that time, we felt that a textbook which brought a number of different research projects in a cohesive form was relevant to the time. This textbook is the result of this effort. It brings together papers from the trainee staff who were part of the Institute of Urology and St Peter's Hospital, many of whom have moved on to their consultant posts since the idea for this book was conceived.

This is a rapidly changing field and inevitably some of the methods of treatment described here have been surpassed. Others remain in everyday use. It has been our intention that the book become a historical record of the state of the art in the late 1980s and early 1990s giving the opportunity to look back to how things were at this time.

I hope that the reader will find the various subjects covered of interest and that the book will find a place on the bookshelf if only to refer to things present and past.

P.J.R. Shah

1 The natural history of benign prostatic hyperplasia

B.C. OGBONA

The natural history of a disease is its prognosis or expected course over time, knowledge of which is necessary for effective therapy. That of benign prostatic hyperplasia (BPH) has not been well studied in the two centuries since this disease was first described (Morgagni, 1760). This is largely because until recently most prostatectomies were absolutely indicated to save life or relieve severe symptoms. But such indications now account for a mere 5 to 10% of the total (Hald, 1989; McKelvie *et al.*, 1993). This and the fact that the number of prostatectomies being performed has risen sharply, with the likelihood in a 40-year-old man increasing from 10% in 1960 to 30% in 1990 (Lytton *et al.*, 1968; Glynn *et al.*, 1985), mean that a large number of relatively indicated operations are being performed, and that the boundaries of clinical disease are as yet very blurred. Before now these relatively indicated operations may have been justified by the assumption that the disease was progressive and early treatment was best (Blandy, 1978). As more information emerges suggesting that this may not necessarily be true (Clarke, 1937; Craigen *et al.*, 1969; Birkhoff *et al.*, 1976; Ball *et al.*, 1981; Barnes & Marsh, 1983; McGuire, 1992), the need for properly controlled studies of the natural history of this disease increases. Adding to this need are the recent concerns about risks and complications of transurethral resection of the prostate (TURP) (Fowler *et al.*, 1988; Roos *et al.*, 1989), its impact on national health budgets (Cockett *et al.*, 1992; McKelvie *et al.*, 1993), as well as the need to evaluate the growing numbers of non-surgical treatment modalities (McGuire, 1992).

The ideal study of the natural history of BPH may involve following into old age a large number of young (<30 years) asymptomatic men, with regular symptom scoring, uroflowmetry, cystometry, and measurements of residual urine and prostatic size. Such a study, daunting as it sounds, would establish baselines in these men and then record separately the onset of various abnormalities which, discovered together many years later, may lead to a wrong diagnosis of BPH. An example would be a young man with a physiologically 'abnormal' voiding pattern which worsens slightly but steadily with age, and whose prostate gland enlarges physiologically but does not affect the rate of deterioration of his voiding. In this way true clinical BPH may be identified and its course observed.

There are two studies in which large numbers of young men have been followed up to chronicle the appearance of urinary obstruction. The Veterans Affairs project (Glynn *et al.*, 1985) started in the 1960s with 2280 healthy Boston area volunteers followed up by symptom analysis and physical examination. These two methods have been shown to be inaccurate in diagnosing BPH (Castro *et al.*, 1969). Also in their report of 1985, analysis was limited to the 1948 men who were initially normal, thus probably omitting valuable information. The Baltimore Longitudinal Study of Aging group (Arrighi *et al.*, 1991) followed up 1371 volunteers from 1958 to 1988 with 2-yearly assessments also limited to history and physical findings.

In the absence of the ideal, a hazy yet perhaps useful picture may be obtained by integrating the results of different studies like the pieces of a jigsaw puzzle, albeit with the pieces greatly mismatched by differences in definitions, population characteristics and methodology.

An attempt to study the community-based incidence of BPH among apparently well men has been made by several workers, but most reports give the incidence of prostatism or prostatectomy rather than BPH. Prostatectomy rates are known to vary in different communities by as much as 20% (Wernberg & Gittelsohn, 1982), and do not reflect the true incidence of the disease (McGuire, 1992). The Veterans Affairs report of 1985 found a 78% cumulative incidence of BPH (based on clinical features) in 40-year-old men surviving to 80 (Glynn *et al.*, 1985). Jensen *et al.* (1986) reported a 17% incidence of prostatism among 112 apparently healthy men aged 50 years and above. However, the random sampling method used, the 60% response rate to the study questionnaire (raising the possibility of the occurrence of selection), and the small population size make the results of this study difficult to assess.

In a large study in which the diagnosis of clinical BPH is more encompassing but which unfortunately does not involve follow-up of patients, Garraway *et al.* (1991) found that 25% of 705 'healthy' men aged 40 to 79 years had clinical BPH. This was defined as enlargement of the prostate gland of equivalent weight >20 g in the presence of urinary dysfunction (using a symptom scale adapted from that devised by Fowler *et al.* (1988)) and/or a urinary peak flow rate <15 ml/s and without evidence of malignancy. McKelvie *et al.* (1993) also found a 25% incidence when this population was increased to 1627 men.

The progress of uncomplicated BPH may be studied from observation of untreated men with proven disease, as well as from the placebo arms of drug trials. Regarding the latter, Barry has pointed out the need to differentiate a symptomatic response to placebo from a natural remission of symptoms (Barry, 1990), while McGuire notes that because of unreliability of prostatic symptoms many of the patients in these studies may not have had the disease that the investigators and the project sponsors wished to study (McGuire, 1992). In one of the earliest reports Clarke (1937) described a retrospective series including 36 patients with 'definite' uncomplicated BPH who had remained symptomatically stable or improved after an average of 5 years. Craigen *et al.* (1969) reported that 10% of 123 patients with symptomatic BPH were symptom-free after 4 years and Birkhoff *et al.* (1976) reported a 43% symptomatic improvement and a 25% objective improvement (based on digital measurement of prostatic size, uroflowmetry and residual urine) among 26 men who refused drug treatment and were followed up for 3 years. The only patient followed up for up to 8 years showed an improvement in objective symptoms.

In 1981 Ball *et al.* described 107 men reassessed 5 years after initial presentation with symptomatic BPH. Of these, 53 had been thought to be urodynamically obstructed. Only 10 patients (all obstructed) had required prostatectomy during this period, while 87 (77%) had remained stable or improved symptomatically. There are no separate follow-up data for the obstructed but untreated patients, and the use of a calculated urethral resistance factor (Pves/Q2) to diagnose obstruction has been criticized (International Continence Society, 1980). Finally, Barnes & Marsh (1983) reported that 56% of 208 men were better or the same after about 5 years of follow-up of untreated symptomatic BPH.

The rate of improvement on the placebo arms of drug trials is quoted at between 10 and 76% over a maximum of about 7 months follow-up (Barry, 1990).

Prediction of progression of untreated, uncomplicated BPH has not been as widely studied. Ball showed that no patient with a urine flow rate within 2 SD of normal (equivalent to 13 ml/s at 250 ml bladder volume) had required surgery during the 5 year period of observation. Also, patients who required surgery had larger prostate glands on profilometry (Ball *et al.*, 1981).

The probability of complications in untreated disease as reported in the literature is equally unclear. The 5 year cumulative incidence of acute retention has been calculated as between 4 and 50% (Barry, 1990). There are no known parameters to predict this occurrence, and Birkhoff *et al.* (1976) show that patients presenting with this complication are not necessarily the most symptomatic. It is, therefore, difficult to advise the individual patient on this risk (Barry, 1990).

The outcome following relief of acute retention has been studied by Taube & Gajraj (1989). Twenty-eight per cent of 60 patients were able to void spontaneously, and 65% of these (or 18% of the total) remained asymptomatic or had minor symptoms 6 months later. However, Breum *et al.* (1982) found that 25% of their patients had a similar previous episode, and in 73% retention recurred within a week.

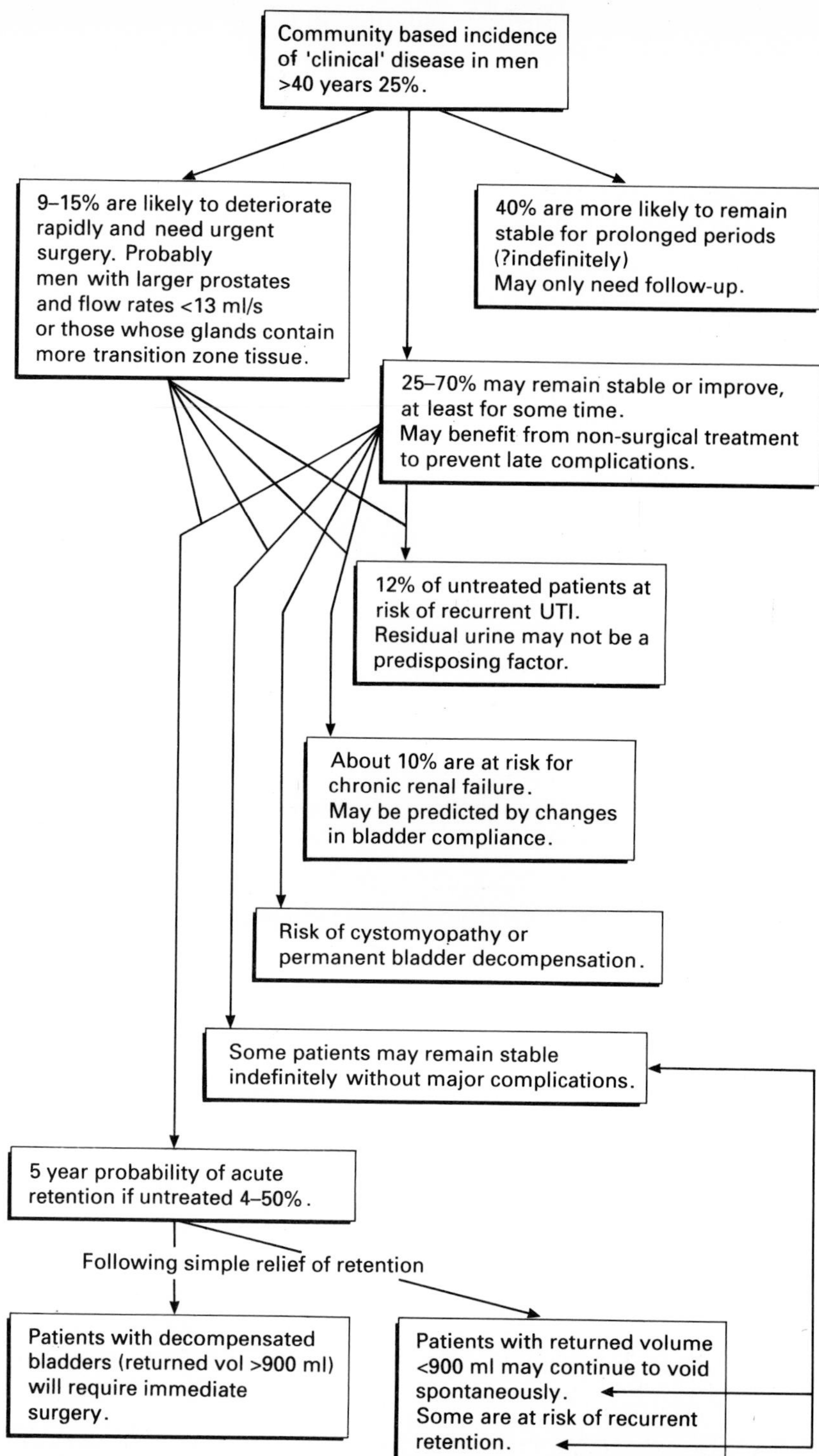

Fig. 1.1. Flow chart to illustrate current knowledge about the natural history of BPH.

Returned volume after relief of retention has been found to be a good predictor of outcome. Fifteen out of 34 patients with <900 ml had a successful voiding trial, while only 2 of 26 patients with >900 ml did (Taube & Gajraj, 1989).

Mebust *et al.* (1989) showed that among 3885 patients undergoing prostatectomy the incidence of recurrent urinary tract infection was 12%. The probability of this complication in men being followed up without treatment is unknown, but a recent study shows that urinary tract infection (UTI) does not always occur in the presence of residual urine (Hampson *et al.*, 1992).

The probability of chronic renal failure is similarly unclear. In one series (Mebust *et al.*, 1989) a serum creatinine >1.5 μg/l was found in 10% of the patients. This complication is dreaded because it may occur in the presence of mild symptoms and produce irreversible damage (Dowd & Ewest, 1961; Beck, 1970). However, changes in bladder compliance may indicate patients at risk from this complication (George *et al.*, 1983; McGuire, 1992). Permanent bladder decompensation or 'cystomyopathy' has been speculated as a consequence of delayed treatment (Barry, 1990). This and the effect of both acute retention and azotemia on the outcome of patients after prostatectomy await proof by randomized clinical trials.

In conclusion, although the natural history of BPH is unknown, a hazy picture emerges from a review of the literature (Fig. 1.1). A clearer picture may appear in the future after the boundaries of clinical disease have been more clearly defined, for which a long period of observation of a large number of asymptomatic young men may be necessary. Clinical BPH probably has no pathological equivalent and may result from a complex interplay of several factors, including a progressive age-related detrusor weakness (probably accounting for the normal deterioration of urine flow rate of about 0.2 ml/s/year (Drach *et al.*, 1979)) and a prostate gland growing normally at the rate of about 0.4 g/year after 30 years of age (Berry *et al.*, 1984), but varying in each individual not only in its rate of growth but also in the proportion of stromal and epithelial tissue contained and hence probably the amount of obstruction produced (McConnell, 1991; Shapiro, 1992).

References

Arrighi H.M., Metler E.J., Guess H.A. & Fozzard J.L. (1991) Natural history of benign prostatic hyperplasia and risk of prostatectomy: the Baltimore Longitudinal Study of Aging. *Urology*, **38** (Suppl. 1), 4–8.

Ball A.J., Feneley R.C.L. & Abrams P.H. (1981) The natural history of untreated 'prostatism'. *Br. J. Urol.*, **53**, 613–16.

Barnes R.W. & Marsh C. (1983) Progression of obstruction and symptoms. In: Hinman F. Jr. (ed.) *Benign Prostatic Hypertrophy*, p. 712. Springer-Verlag, New York.

Barry M.J. (1990) Epidemiology and natural history of benign prostatic hyperplasia. *Urol. Clin. N. Amer.*, **17**(3), 495–507.

Beck D. (1970) Benign prostatic hyperplasia and uremia. A review of 315 cases. *Br. J. Surg.*, **57**, 561–5.

Berry S.J., Coffey D.S. & Walsh P.C. (1984) The development of human BPH with age. *J. Urol.*, **132**, 474–9.

Birkhoff J.D., Wiederhorn A.R., Hamilton M.C. & Zinsser H.H. (1976) Natural history of benign prostatic hypertrophy and acute urinary retention. *Urology*, **7**, 48–52.

Blandy J.P. (1978) The indications for prostatectomy. *Urol. Int.*, **33**, 159–70.

Breum L., Klaoskov P., Munck L.K., Nielson T.H. & Nordestgaard A.G. (1982) Significance of acute urinary retention due to intravesical obstruction. *Scand. J. Urol. Nephrol.*, **16**, 21–4.

Castro J.E., Griffiths A.J.L. & Shackman R. (1969) Significance of signs and symptoms in BPH. *Br. Med. J.*, **2**, 598–601.

Clarke R. (1937) The prostate and the endocrines. A control series. *Br. J. Urol.*, **9**, 254–71.

Cockett A.T.K., Barry M.J., Holtgrew H.L., Sihelnick S., Williams R. & McConnell J. (1992) Indications for treatment of benign prostatic hyperplasia. *Cancer*, **70** (Suppl. 1), 280–3.

Craigen A.A., Hickling J.B. & Saunders C.R. (1969) Natural history of prostatic obstruction. A prospective study. *J. Roy. Coll. Gen. Pract.*, **18**, 226–32.

Dowd J.B. & Ewest E.E. (1961) Silent prostatism (unrecognised bladder neck obstruction). *JAMA*, **178**, 296–300.

Drach G.W., Layton T.N. & Binard W.J. (1979) Male peak urinary flow rates: relationship to voided volume and age. *J. Urol.*, **122**, 210–14.

Fowler F.J. Jr., Wennberg J.E., Timothy R.P., Barry M.J., Mulley A.G. Jr. & Hanley D. (1988) Symptom status and quality of life following prostatectomy. *JAMA*, **259**, 3018–22.

Garraway W.M., Collins G.N. & Lee R.J. (1991) High prevalence of benign prostatic hypertrophy in the community. *Lancet*, **338**, 469–71.

George N.J.R., O'Reilly P.H., Barnard R.J. & Blacklock N.J. (1983) High pressure chronic retention. *Br. Med. J.*, **286**, 1780–3.

Glynn R.J., Campion E.W., Bouchard G.R. & Silbert J.E. (1985) The development of benign prostatic hyperplasia among volunteers in the normative ageing study. *Am. J. Epidemiol.*, **121**, 78–90.

Hald T. (1989) Urodynamics in benign prostatic hyperplasia: a survey. *Prostate*, **2** (Suppl.), 69–77.

Hampson A.J., Noble J.G., Rickards D. & Milroy E.J.G. (1992) Does residual urine predispose to urinary tract infection? *Br. J. Urol.*, **70**, 506–8.

International Continence Society. (1980) Third report on the standardisation of terminology of lower urinary tract function. *Br. J. Urol.*, **52**, 348–50.

Jensen K.M.E., Jorgensen J.B., Morgensen P. & Bille-Brahe N.E. (1986) Some clinical aspects of uroflowmetry in elderly males: a population study. *Scand. J. Urol. Nephrol.*, **20**, 93–7.

Lytton B., Emery J.M. & Harvard B.M. (1968) The incidence of benign prostate obstruction. *J. Urol.*, **99**, 638–45.

McConnell J.D. (1991) The pathophysiology of benign prostatic hyperplasia. *J. Androl.*, **12**, 356–63.

McGuire E.J. (1992) The role of urodynamic investigation in the assessment of benign prostatic hypertrophy. *J. Urol.*, **148**, 1133–6.

McKelvie G.B., Collins G.N., Hehir M. & Rogers A.C.N. (1993) A study of benign prostatic hyperplasia: a challenge to British urology. *Br. J. Urol.*, **71**, 38–42.

Mebust W.K., Holtgrew H.L. & Cockett A.T. (1989) Transurethral prostatectomy: immediate and postoperative complications. A co-operative study of 13 participating institutions evaluating 3885 patients. *J. Urol.*, **141**, 243–7.

Morgagni G.B. (1760) *The Seats and Causes of Disease Investigated by Anatomy*, Book 3, p. 460. Johnson & Paine, London.

Roos N.P., Wennberg J.E., Malenka D.J., Fisher E.S., McPherson K., Anderson T.F., Cohen M.M. & Ramsey E. (1989) Mortality and reoperation after open and transurethral resection of the prostate for benign prostatic hyperplasia. *New Engl. J. Med.*, **320**, 1120–4.

Shapiro E. (1992) The relative proportion of stromal and epithelial hyperplasia is related to the development of symptomatic BPH. *J. Urol.*, **147**, 1293–7.

Taube M. & Gajraj H. (1989) Trial without catheter following acute retention of urine. *Br. J. Urol.*, **63**, 180–2.

Wernberg J. & Gittelsohn A. (1982) Variations in medical care among small areas. *Sci. Am.*, **246**, 100–11.

2 The diagnosis of prostatic outflow obstruction

P.J.R. SHAH

Introduction

Benign enlargement of the prostate affects the majority of the male population as they age. It has been reported that 50% of males over the age of 65 years have symptoms consistent with a diagnosis of prostatic outflow obstruction (Lytton *et al.*, 1968) with up to 500 000 men in the UK with symptoms that interfere with daily activities. McKelvie *et al.* (1992) also showed that of 1627 eligible men in the 40–79 year age group (the ineligible men had been excluded because of a history of previous urinary tract surgery or spinal disease) 34.5% were found to have symptoms relating to the bladder or low measured urinary flow rate. Approximately one in four men in the population have measurable benign prostatic enlargement (Garraway *et al.*, 1991). This figure may be even greater than 25%. In a study of 1057 men followed for up to 30 years 49.8% were found to have clinically diagnosed benign prostatic hyperplasia (BPH) (Arrighi *et al.*, 1991). Thus, the problem of the management of symptomatic prostatic outflow obstruction with an increase in the ageing male population promises to be immense. The importance of having as much information about the natural history of the disease is paramount.

We need to know not only the prevalence of the disease but also:

- The consequences of prostatic outflow obstruction on bladder function.
- The consequences of outflow obstruction on renal function.
- The likely incidence of the development of retention.
- The success rate of surgical treatment in comparison with a watch-and-wait policy.
- The use of the new methods of treatment of prostatic outflow obstruction.
- The risk of missing prostatic carcinoma.

Symptoms of prostatic outflow obstruction

Narrowing of the prostatic urethra which is a consequence of enlargement of the prostate produces a number of symptoms which usually develop gradually in the ageing male. The symptoms are due to changes in the dynamics of bladder function but are not always explained by the simple analogy of obstruction to the outflow. McConnell (1991) states that 'a significant portion of the symptoms are due to obstruction induced detrusor dysfunction. . .and neural alterations in the bladder'.

In dynamic terms the natural history of prostatic obstruction may be such that the following occurs:

normal function: normal pressure/normal flow
early obstruction: high pressure/normal flow
established obstruction: high pressure/low flow
decompensated obstruction: low pressure/low flow
retention either acute, chronic or acute on chronic.

Each of these stages may be asymptomatic for a particular male except the onset of retention of urine. However, symptoms will tend to become more apparent and troublesome the greater the effects of obstruction on the bladder.

Symptoms tend to fall into two separate categories. For the purposes of diagnosis and treatment of prostatic obstruction, these two categories are separated for good reason:

1. Pure symptoms of outflow obstruction

Hesitancy: having to wait before flow starts. This delay is probably due to a combination of factors which are related to the higher pressures that are needed to produce flow and delay in the initiation of the voiding reflex.

Poor stream: a reduction in the urinary flow is a consequence of compression of the prostatic urethra and the inability of the detrusor muscle to reach a sufficiently high pressure to maintain flow at its normal level.

This sequence of events may occur in all normal males who are developing outflow obstruction. It is likely that the degree of obstruction will vary from individual to individual and that a status quo may be reached in an individual that does not progress to a point at which surgical treatment is necessary. There is evidence that little change in voiding parameters takes place in established obstruction over a number of months (Kadow *et al.*, 1988) or years (Ball *et al.*, 1981). Predicting those patients that will inevitably develop the more serious consequences of high-pressure chronic retention (Abrams & Feneley, 1978) or large-capacity low-pressure chronic retention has not yet been possible. Though Styles *et al.* (1991) suggest that the main risk factors for upper tract dilatation are 'a pressure increase during bladder filling and the frequency of phasic detrusor activity during long-term monitoring'.

Terminal dribbling (TD) is a common symptom in males with obstruction. When voiding has come near to completion, urine still flows but very slowly as a dribble. This TD takes place before the completion of voiding and must be differentiated from post-micturition dribbling (PMD) which occurs after micturition has been completed and is urine draining from the horizontal portion of the bulbar urethra. PMD gives rise to wetting of the underclothing, a distressing symptom for some males. This symptom is not associated with prostatic obstruction. It occurs from time to time in all normal males though some individuals are more troubled than others. Occasionally, PMD indicates a urethral stricture or urethral diverticulum.

Retention of urine whether acute or chronic is a symptom of prostatic outflow obstruction though it may be caused by a urethral stricture and many other less common causes.

2. *Irritative symptoms*

Irritative symptoms are commonly associated with prostatic outflow obstruction (Abrams *et al.*, 1978; Sibley, 1985). Prostatic outflow obstruction causes bladder instability. Approximately 65% of males with prostatic obstruction will have associated bladder instability. The symptoms are:

Frequency of micturition: passing urine frequently — more than seven times a day (depending upon fluid intake).

Urgency: a feeling of urgent need to void. This symptom is due to unstable detrusor contractions.

Urge incontinence: associated with the urgent need to pass urine (incontinence may occur). When studied urodynamically, it is very high-pressure detrusor contractions that give rise to urge incontinence, when the unstable detrusor pressure exceeds the outflow resistance. Urge incontinence is, however, not as common in the male with instability as it is in the female whose urethra does not exert such a high pressure.

Nocturia: being awoken by the desire to void at night is left to last in this group of symptoms even though it is often the symptom that is most troublesome to the patient. Nocturia is common in the elderly due to a number of non-obstructive factors:

- Poor sleeping habits
- Fluid redistribution after peripheral pooling of fluid during the day
- A change in the diurnal regulation of fluid output
- Habit
- Inappropriate drinking
- Bladder instability

Before nocturia as the predominant symptom may be attributed to outflow obstruction the above factors should be considered.

A *frequency/volume voided chart* (Table 2.1) will be a useful guide as to some of these factors and a rearrangement of fluid intake alone may improve some symptoms.

Symptom scores

Do symptom scores predict the most severely obstructed patients? Do symptom scores help to indicate the likely outcome of treatment and can they be effectively used for the selection of patients for treatment?

Symptom score charts have gained in popularity since they were first described by Boyarsky *et al.* (1977) and Madsen & Iverson (1983). There is no doubt that a symptom scoring system is useful in quantifying the degree of 'suffering' with prostatic symptoms. A symptom scoring system has recently been devised by the American Urological Association (Table 2.2). It may be that the irritative symptoms that are associated with prostatic outflow obstruction may require heavier weighting, since they are more troublesome to the patient and produce greater patient satisfaction if they are relieved, than the pure obstructive symptoms.

A visual analogue scale (Table 2.3) has been found of use in assessing whether low flow rates were due to obstruction or poor detrusor contractility (McLoughlin *et al.*, 1990).

Although symptom scores are of benefit in aiding diagnosis they still require confirmation by urodynamic study in one form or another. If a patient's symptoms improve over a period of months there is little likelihood of retention of urine developing (Nohr *et al.*, 1991).

Investigations

Can we select patients for surgery on the basis of non-invasive tests or should all patients undergo urodynamic study?

After the clinical history has been taken (a proforma on which to record the history (Table 2.4) is most useful or a symptom score chart or both) a clinical examination should be performed. Abdominal examination to detect a palpable bladder or other masses should be followed by a rectal examination. The size and consistency of the prostate should be recorded. Measurement of prostatic specific antigen (PSA) appears justified in patients with prostatic outflow obstruction (Powell *et al.*, 1989). If the prostate feels hard or nodular, prostatic ultrasound scanning is recommended. The size of the prostate has relevance to the type of treatment, particularly surgery, but does not relate to the degree of obstruction.

A mid-stream urine should be collected for examination for cells and culture. An abdominal radiograph is not essential but may be indicated if

Table 2.1. Frequency/volume chart

Name .... **Record number** ....
Date of start ....

	Sunday		Monday		Tuesday		Wednesday		Thursday		Friday		Saturday	
	IN	OUT	IN	OUT	IN	OUT	IN	OUT	IN	OUT	IN	OUT	IN	OUT
09.00–10.00														
10.00–11.00														
11.00–12.00														
12.00–13.00														
13.00–14.00														
14.00–15.00														
15.00–16.00														
16.00–17.00														
17.00–18.00														
18.00–19.00														
19.00–20.00														
20.00–21.00														
21.00–22.00														
22.00–23.00														
23.00–24.00														
24.00–01.00														
01.00–02.00														
02.00–03.00														
03.00–04.00														
04.00–05.00														
05.00–06.00														
06.00–07.00														
07.00–08.00														
08.00–09.00														
Waking														
Retiring														

Enter amount drunk in the 'in' column. Enter volumes of urine passed in the 'out' column. Please return this completed chart at your next visit.

Table 2.2. Symptom scoring system (American Urological Association)

Lower urinary tract symptoms score **Name**

Please read this questionnaire and circle or tick the number of whichever description most closely describes each of your symptoms. Please bring the form with you to discuss with me in the outpatient clinic.

Obstructive symptoms		**Description**
Hesitancy	0	Occasional (occurs in less than 20% of attempts to void)
	1	Moderate (occurs in 20–50% of attempts to void)
	2	Frequent (occurs in more than 50% of attempts to void but not always and may last up to 1 minute)
	3	Always present and lasts for more than 1 minute
Intermittency	0	Occasional (occurs in less than 20% of attempts to void)
	1	Moderate (occurs in 20–50% of attempts to void)
	2	Frequent (occurs in more than 50% of attempts to void but not always and may last up to 1 minute)
	3	Always present and lasts for more than 1 minute
Terminal dribbling	0	Occasional (occurs in less than 20% of attempts to void)
	1	Moderate (occurs in 20–50% of attempts to void)
	2	Frequent (occurs in more than 50% of attempts to void but not always)
	3	Always present and lasts for more than 1 minute or wets clothing
Impairment of stream	0	Absence of symptoms
	1	Impaired trajectory, i.e. 'Does not hit the wall like it used to'
	2	Most of the time size and force are restricted
	3	Patient urinates with great effort and the stream is interrupted
Sense of emptying	0	Absence of symptom
	1	Occasional sensation of incomplete bladder emptying after voiding
	2	Frequent (more than 50% of the time) sensation of incomplete bladder emptying after voiding
	3	Constant and urgent sensation and no relief upon voiding
	15	

(continued)

Table 2.2. (continued)

Irritative symptoms		
Nocturia	0	Absence of symptom
	1	Patient awakens once each night to urinate
	2	Patient awakens 2–3 times each night to urinate
	3	Patient awakens more than 4 times each night to urinate
Daytime frequency	0	Patient urinates 1–4 times daily
	1	Patient urinates 5–7 times daily
	2	Patient urinates 8–12 times daily
	3	Patient urinates more than 13 times daily
Urgency	0	Absence of symptom
	1	Occasionally difficult for patient to postpone urination
	2	Frequently difficult (more than 50% of the time) to postpone urination and may rarely lose urine
	3	Always difficult to postpone urination and may sometimes lose urine
Dysuria	0	Absence of symptom
	1	Occasional burning sensation during urination
	2	Frequently (more than 50% of the time) a burning sensation during urination
	3	Frequent and painful burning sensation during urination
	12	
Max score	**27**	

Please add any comments you wish to make here ....
....

there are upper urinary tract symptoms or symptoms suggestive of calculus anywhere in the urinary tract. Urinary tract ultrasound may be performed but is not essential in every patient, though a justification may be made for its use in all patients because of its simplicity and non-invasion.

A free urine flow rate is essential in all patients with prostatic outflow obstruction, several flow rates being preferable in a flow rate clinic. The patient should have a comfortably full bladder, not overfull. An overfull bladder will affect the urine flow rate adversely.

A post-micturition ultrasound scan of the bladder will demonstrate whether residual urine is present. Thus, flowmetry and ultrasonography are ideally combined.

Table 2.3. A visual analogue scale
(a) Urinary symptoms

	Not at all	Less than 1 time in 5	Less than half the time	About half the time	More than half the time	Almost always
1. Over the past month or so, how often have you had a sensation of not emptying your bladder completely after you finished urinating?	0	1	2	3	4	5
2. Over the past month or so, how often have you had to urinate again less than two hours after you finished urinating?	0	1	2	3	4	5
3. Over the past month or so, how often have you found you stopped and started again several times when urinating?	0	1	2	3	4	5
4. Over the past month or so, how often have you found it difficult to postpone urination?	0	1	2	3	4	5
5. Over the past month or so, how often have you had a weak urinary stream?	0	1	2	3	4	5
6. Over the past month or so, how often have you had to push or strain to begin urination?	0	1	2	3	4	5
7. Over the last month, how many times did you most typically get up to urinate from the time you went to bed at night until the time you got up in the morning? (0 = none, 1 = 1 time, 2 = 2 times, 3 = 3 times, 4 = 4 times, 5 = 5 or more times)						

Urodynamic investigations

Cystometry or videocystometry where available are the best methods of confirming outflow obstruction. The pressure/flow rate study will usually be able to demonstrate obstruction, high pressure/reduced flow being the measure by which obstruction is diagnosed on urodynamics. The filling cystometrogram will demonstrate whether bladder instability is present. If synchronous radiological screening is available (video) the bladder neck and prostatic urethra may be seen.

Table 2.3. (continued)
(b) Problems due to symptoms

	No problem	Very small problem	Small problem	Medium problem	Big problem
1. Over the past month, how much has a sensation of not emptying your bladder been a problem for you?	0	1	2	3	4
2. Over the past month has frequent urination during the day been a problem to you?	0	1	2	3	4
3. Over the past month how much has getting up at night to urinate been a problem for you?	0	1	2	3	4
4. Over the past month, how much has stopping and starting when you urinate been a problem for you?	0	1	2	3	4
5. Over the past month, how much has a need to urinate with little warning been a problem for you?	0	1	2	3	4
6. Over the past month, how much have impaired size and force of urinary stream been a problem for you?	0	1	2	3	4
7. Over the past month how much has having to push or strain to begin urination been a problem for you?	0	1	2	3	4

Compression of the prostatic urethra is pathognomonic of obstruction. However, bladder-neck obstruction should be distinguished from prostatic obstruction. Bladder-neck obstruction on 'video' is confirmed by failure of the bladder neck to open in early voiding, though it usually opens later in voiding. Trapping of contrast between the bladder neck and external sphincter during the 'stop test' at the point of maximum flow is pathognomonic of bladder neck obstruction (Whiteside sign) (Bates *et al.*, 1970).

Ambulatory urodynamic studies are useful when results from cystometry are equivocal. This particularly applies to incomplete studies in which

Table 2.4. Proforma to record history of patient

<table>
<tr><td colspan="2">NAME . . . . DATE OF BIRTH . . . GP . . .
ADDRESS . . . . AGE . . . .
. . . .
POSTCODE . . . . TEL . . . .</td></tr>
<tr><td colspan="2">PRESENTING COMPLAINT</td></tr>
<tr><td>Frequency
Nocturia
Urgency
Incontinence — urge/stress
— continuous
— unconscious
Enuresis

Hesitancy
Stream
Straining
TD — PMD
Incomplete emptying

Dysuria
Infection
Haematuria
Pain — loin — urethral — bladder
— elsewhere</td><td rowspan="5">Investigations

Management</td></tr>
<tr><td>Sexual function
— erection
— ejaculation
— frequency</td></tr>
<tr><td>Past medical history</td></tr>
<tr><td>Family history

Drugs Allergies</td></tr>
<tr><td rowspan="2">Examination

Pelvic — rectal

Diagnosis</td></tr>
<tr><td>Date Operations</td></tr>
</table>

either the pressure catheters fall out during the voiding phase of the study or when the patient finds it difficult to void during the study. Ambulatory studies should be performed using a fine suprapubic catheter or micro-tip transducer catheter which will not fall out during voiding.

Pressure/flow plots and nomograms may help to diagnose obstruction when the results are equivocal.

Urethral pressure profilometry (UPP) no longer has a place in the routine clinical diagnosis of prostatic outflow obstruction. However, UPP is a useful investigation in clinical trials of therapeutic regimens.

Do the new computer-generated assessments of bladder function help to predict those patients that may respond to treatment?

There is some evidence that computer-aided programmes, e.g. CLIM (Rollema *et al.*, 1991), will provide reliable information about obstruction and contractility parameters.

Endoscopy

Cystourethroscopy should be performed prior to prostatic surgery. However, a diagnosis of prostatic outflow obstruction should not be made on a cystoscopic inspection alone. A dynamic test of voiding function, flow rate +/− cystometry should be performed prior to endoscopy.

Conclusion

When a patient presents with symptoms suggestive of prostatic outflow obstruction two important facts must be considered: is the prostate benign and is obstruction present? A clinical history using symptom score charts, an abdominal and rectal examination and dynamic study of bladder function must be performed to provide a correct diagnosis. Additional investigations may be necessary in order to validate the diagnosis. It seems illogical to perform a surgical procedure with all its attendant risks when urodynamic investigations may be carried out with minimal morbidity both quickly and inexpensively. Many otherwise unnecessary operations may be avoided. An understanding of the natural history of prostatic obstruction is, however, fundamental to the management of this common condition. If we were able to predict those patients who could be safely left without treatment, without detriment to bladder and upper tracts, this could save much surgical intervention. We should also be able to predict those patients who would be best served by drug therapy, microwave treatment or

PROSTATE INFORMATION SHEET

The Prostate is a gland situated around the outlet of the bladder in men.

PROSTATE

The main symptoms of an enlarged prostate are:

- delay in passing urine.
- poor flow.
- dribbling.
- a feeling of incomplete bladder emptying.

With age, the prostate may grow and constrict the bladder outflow leading to difficulty passing urine.

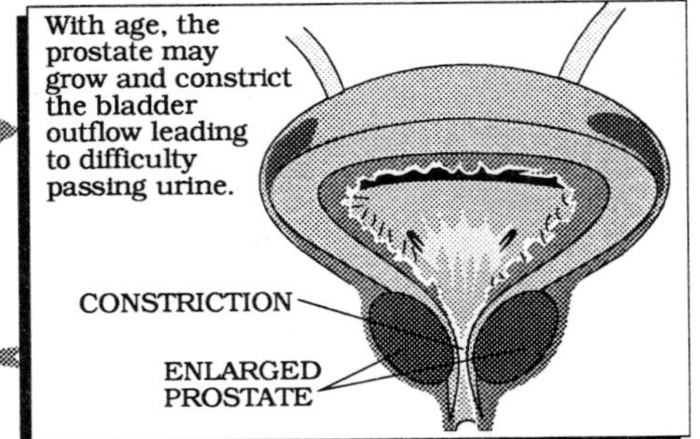

DIAGNOSIS

After referral to a hospital specialist certain examination and tests may be undertaken to assess the amount of prostate enlargement and obstruction.

EXAMINATION OF THE PROSTATE
The Doctor will be able to obtain a lot of information by directly feeling the gland.

FLOW TEST
You will be asked to pass water into a special machine which measures urine flow. You need to pass at least 200mls for the test to be readable, so come to each clinic visit prepared with a full bladder.

X-RAY AND ULTRASOUND SCAN
These will check the kidneys and bladder and show how much urine is being 'left-behind' in the bladder after urinating.

A SPECIAL SCAN OF THE PROSTATE (TRUS)
This can give a more detailed picture of the prostate. It involves passing a small scanner into the back passage which can see the prostate directly.

A BLOOD TEST
The blood test checks the kidney function and also measures a special substance exclusively produced by the prostate.

THE TREATMENT

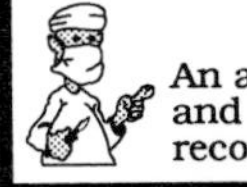

An assessment of the degree of obstruction, size of the prostate and a check to exclude cancer will now have been made. The recommended options will be discussed at this stage.

WAIT AND SEE
A proportion of patients will have symptoms they can live with, which do not interfere with daily life and on testing the obstruction is minor.

TABLETS
A number of drugs are available to help either shrink the prostate or relax it. These drugs are unsuited to certain patients but may prove extremely beneficial to some.

OPERATIONS
The standard operation on the prostate is the 'TURP' or transurethral resection. It has evolved over many years and is an effective and safe procedure. Most patients stay in hospital only 5 days, and as the operation is performed using a telescope through the penis, there are no scars. Occasionally, if the prostate is very large, an open operation is performed instead.

STENTS
In people who are felt to be at risk from a full prostate operation, as a result of ill health, metal 'stents' can be placed internally, under local anaesthetic, to hold the bladder outlet open.

NEW TREATMENTS
Lasers, Microwaves and enhanced ultrasound are all currently being assessed as an alternative to operation. Long term results of these techniques are awaited.

Fig. 2.1. Prostate information sheet.

surgery. If this were possible, selected treatments for individuals would also be possible.

Providing the patient with information is also very important so that he recognizes the nature of both investigation and treatment. We use a prostate information sheet (Fig. 2.1) for patient education in our centre which helps to explain the various investigations and treatment methods and allows a patient to make a better-informed decision about which treatment policy is preferable and subsequently chosen for him.

References

Abrams P.H. & Feneley R.C.L. (1978) The significance of symptoms associated with bladder outflow obstruction. *Urol. Int.*, **33**, 171–4.

Abrams P.H., Dunn M. & George N. (1978) Urodynamic findings in chronic retention of urine and their relevance to results of surgery. *Br. Med. J.*, **2**, 1258–60.

Arrighi H.M., Metter E.J., Guess H.A. & Fozzard J.L. (1991) Natural history of benign prostatic hyperplasia and risk of prostatectomy. The Baltimore Longitudinal Study of Aging. *Urology*, **38** (Suppl. 1), 4–8.

Ball A.J., Feneley R.C.L. & Abrams P.H. (1981) The natural history of prostatism. *Br. J. Urol.*, **53**, 613–6.

Bates C.P., Whiteside C.G. & Turner-Warwick R.T. (1970) Synchronous video pressure flow cysto-urethrography. *Br. J. Urol.*, **42**, 714–22.

Boyarsky S., Jones G., Paulson D.F. & Prout G.R. Jr. (1977) A new look at bladder neck obstruction by the Food and Drug Administration Regulators: guidelines for the investigation of benign prostatic hypertrophy. *Transamerican Assoc. Genitourinary Surg.*, **68**, 29–32.

Garraway W.M., Collins G.N. & Lee R.J. (1991) High prevalence of benign prostatic hypertrophy in the community. *Lancet*, **338**(8765), 469–71.

Kadow C., Feneley R.C. & Abrams P.H. (1988) Prostatectomy or conservative management in the treatment of benign prostatic hypertrophy? *Br. J. Urol.*, **61**, 432–4.

Lytton B., Emery J.M. & Harvard B.M. (1968) The incidence of benign prostatic hypertrophy. *Transamerican Assoc. Genitourinary Surg.*, **59**, 65–71.

McConnell J.D. (1991) The pathophysiology of benign prostatic hyperplasia. *J. Androl.*, **12**, 356–63.

McKelvie G.B., Collins G.N., Hehir M. & Rogers A.C.N. (1992) A study of benign prostatic hyperplasia. A challenge to British urology. *Br. J. Urol.*, **71**, 38–42.

McLoughlin J., Abel P.D., Shaikh N., Waters J. & Williams G. (1990) Visual analogue scales distinguish between low urinary flow rates due to impaired detrusor contractility and those due to bladder outflow obstruction. *Br. J. Urol.*, **66**, 16–18.

Madsen P.O. & Iverson P.A. (1983) A point scoring system for selecting operative candidates. In: Hinman F. Jr. & Boyarski S. (eds) *Benign Prostatic Hypertrophy*, pp. 763–9. Springer-Verlag, New York.

Neal D.E., Styles R.A., Powell P.H., Thong J. & Ramsden P.D. (1987) Relationship between voiding pressures, symptoms and urodynamic findings in 253 men undergoing prostatectomy. *Br. J. Urol.*, **60**, 554–9.

Nohr S.B., Jensen B.N., Mortensen B.B. & Walter S. (1991) Prostatic hypertrophy: natural history. Subjective and objective changes during a 6 month period. *Ugeskr-Laeger*, **153**, 1474–7.

Powell C.S., Fielding A.M., Rosser K., Ames A.C. & Vaughton K.C. (1989) Prostatic specific antigen — a screening test for prostatic cancer. *Br. J. Urol.*, **64**, 504–6.

Rollema H.J., van Mastrigt R. & Janknegt R.A. (1991) Urodynamic assessment and quantification of prostatic obstruction before and after transurethral resection of the prostate: standardization with the aid of the computer program CLIM. *Urol. Int.*, **47** (Suppl. 1), 52–4.

Sibley G.N.A. (1985) An experimental model of detrusor instability in the obstructed pig. *Br. J. Urol.*, **57**, 292–8.

Speakman M.J., Sethia K.K., Fellows G.J. & Smith J.C. (1987) A study of the pathogenesis, urodynamic assessment and outcome of detrusor instability associated with bladder outflow obstruction. *Br. J. Urol.*, **59**, 40–4.

Styles R.A., Ramsden P.D. & Neal D.E. (1991) The outcome of prostatectomy on chronic retention of urine. *J. Urol.*, **146**, 1029–33.

3 Medical management of prostatic outflow obstruction

G. DAS

Introduction

The surgical treatment of prostatic outflow obstruction, whether by transurethral prostatectomy or open operation, has long been well established. Surgery gives good results in the majority of patients, especially when correctly selected for those with proven bladder outlet obstruction. However, there are morbidity and mortality associated with prostatic surgery as indeed there are with any form of surgical intervention.

Therefore, the search for non-surgical means of treatment of benign prostatic hyperplasia (BPH) has progressed, and in recent years several pharmacological options have come to light. This chapter outlines the various drug treatments currently available, the scientific basis of their use, the results of clinical trials, and the role of drugs in the treatment of BPH. The various medical agents used in BPH can be categorized as follows:

- alpha-adrenergic antagonists
- 5-alpha-reductase inhibitors
- anti-androgens and aromatase inhibitors
- GnRH (gonadotrophin-releasing hormone) agonists
- natural plant extracts.

Alpha-adrenergic antagonists

Rationale for use

Morphological studies by Bartsch *et al.* (1979) showed that, although the prostate is considered to be a glandular structure, it also contains a large amount of fibromuscular stroma. By performing electron microscopic stereometric analysis they were able to show that in BPH the percentage of the stromal element significantly increased to about 60% as compared with 45% in the normal gland. This anatomical finding led to the suggestion that BPH arises largely by stromal overgrowth. It was also generally accepted that bladder outflow obstruction resulting from benign prostatic enlargement was due to two factors: a static anatomical element due to the physical mass of the adenoma; and a dynamic neuro-pharmacologically mediated component which was the tone of the smooth muscle in the stromal tissue of the prostate and the prostatic capsule causing functional compression of the prostatic urethra. Early studies by Caine *et al.* (1975) on the receptor content of BPH had indicated that large numbers of alpha-adrenergic receptors were present in the smooth muscle of the adenoma and also in the prostatic capsule. It was also shown that alpha-receptor stimulation of the smooth muscle component of BPH, both in the adenoma and capsule, caused increased muscle tone.

Subsequent studies by Chapple *et al.* (1989) further characterized this adrenergic stromal innervation. They demonstrated a functional and ultrastructural preponderance of alpha-1-receptors over alpha-2-receptors in the stromal tissue. These academic studies, along with the clinical observation by Thien *et al.* (1987) that treatment of hypertension with the selective alpha-blocker prazosin led to urinary incontinence in women, paved the way for clinical trials in the use of alpha-blockers for prostatic obstruction.

Clinical trials with alpha-blockers

The various alpha-blockers which have been used in clinical practice include:

- phenoxybenzamine
- prazosin
- indoramin
- terazosin
- Alfuzosin
- YM 617
- Doxazosin.

Phenoxybenzamine The earliest alpha-agonist to be used in clinical trials was phenoxybenzamine. In the first double-blind, placebo-controlled trial, Caine *et al.* (1978) using 10 mg of phenoxybenzamine twice daily for 2 weeks reported an average increase in voiding peak flow by 6.2 ml/s compared with 1.2 ml/s in the placebo group. Symptomatic improvement was also documented in the treated group. Other studies have supported these results. Boreham *et al.* (1977), in their uncontrolled study, demonstrated symptomatic improvement in the majority at the expense of side-effects which occurred in two-thirds of patients. Abrams *et al.* (1982) also showed improvement with 10 mg (twice daily for 4 weeks) in a total of 41 patients. However, Brooks *et al.* (1983) and Ferrie & Paterson (1986) were unable to demonstrate any benefit. Alpha-blockade has also been shown to be of use in acute retention and also for prophylaxis against acute retention.

Phenoxybenzamine produces side-effects due to the fact that it is a non-selective adrenoceptive agonist, i.e. it blocks alpha-receptors on the target smooth muscle cell as well as the alpha-2-receptors on the parent nerve cell. This negates the alpha-2-adrenoceptor-mediated feedback control of noradrenaline. The side-effects produced such as postural hypotension, reflex tachycardia, dizziness, nasal congestion and retrograde ejaculation are thus due to excess noradrenaline release.

At the time of writing, discussion of the clinical use of phenoxybenzamine is academic as recent animal experiments have suggested that phenoxybenzamine could be mutagenic and it is therefore unavailable for general clinical use in the United Kingdom. A scrutiny of the trials using phenoxybenzamine is, however, important, as these trials established, for the first time, clinical usefulness of an adrenoceptive agent while drawing attention to the limitations of use due to side-effects and also poor results when compared with transurethral prostatectomy.

As already mentioned many of the side-effects of phenoxybenzamine were ascribed to its non-selective adrenoceptive effect. To try and reduce the side-effects, attempts were made to use selective alpha-blockers to treat BPH. The following agents are all alpha-blockers and have been extensively used in clinical trials.

Prazosin Prazosin is a highly selective alpha-blocker. Early trials by Hedlund *et al.* (1983) and Martorana *et al.* (1984) were placebo-controlled with small numbers of patients. Both studies showed significantly increased voiding flow rates in the treatment group. The effects on symptom scores were more difficult to assess, partly due to the significant placebo effects commonly observed in the non-operative treatment of BPH. Kirby *et al.* (1987) reported a trial in which 80 patients were entered. There were 25 withdrawals or exclusions, leaving 55 patients for analysis. Of these, 28 were treated with prazosin while 27 received placebo. Over a period of 4 weeks, patients received escalating doses of prazosin commencing with a dose of 500 μg b.d. to 2 mg b.d. Results were judged according to the urodynamic criteria of end fill pressure and voiding peak flow rate, residual volume and symptomatic assessment of frequency and nocturia. Kirby *et al.* (1987) found an increase in peak flow rate from 8 ml to 13 ml/s in the treated group and also statistically significant improvement in irritative symptoms. Interestingly, side-effects were found to be similar in both groups and there were no detectable effects of prazosin on either erect or supine blood pressure. No patient in either group complained of ejaculatory dysfunction or erectile failure.

Indoramin Indoramin is a competitive alpha-adrenoceptor antagonist with no beta-blocking or anti-cholinergic properties. An initial study by Iacovou and Dunn (1987) using doses of 50 and 100 mg daily of indoramin produced significant symptomatic improvement and increased peak flow rates. A further study by Stott and Abrams (1991) demonstrated improved peak flow rate and reduced nocturia at the better tolerated dose of 20 mg twice daily. These encouraging results led to the setting up of a large multi-centre double-blind placebo-controlled trial (Chow *et al.*, 1990). A total of 139 patients suffering from symptoms of bladder outlet obstruction due to BPH were entered into the trial. They were randomly allocated into three groups to receive either placebo, indoramin 20 mg nocte or indoramin 20 mg twice daily. They returned at 4 and 8 weeks and assessment by way of symptom scores and flow rates was performed. There were 18 withdrawals or exclusions leaving 121 patients for analysis. Results showed that 78% of patients taking indoramin 20 mg b.d. reported symptomatic improvement compared with 64% of those taking indoramin 20 mg once daily and 53% of those taking placebo. The physician's assessment of improvement in symptom was 76%, 63% and 30% respectively ($P > 0.01$). When peak flow rates were analysed there was increase of peak flow by 4.9 ml/s in the 20 mg b.d. group ($P > 0.01$).

Terazosin The primary advantage of terazosin over other alpha-blockers is that it has a longer half-life which permits dosing of once a day. In an early study by Lepor *et al.* (1990) 45 normotensive men with symptomatic BPH were treated with a dose of terazosin titrated to 5 mg/day over a course of 1 month. Results were determined on the basis of urinary peak flow rates and symptom scores. The peak and mean urinary flow rates improved by 42% and 48% respectively. Obstructive and irritative symptoms improved by 63% and 45% respectively. Both were statistically significant. Only one patient developed significant hypotension. Overall, there were insignificant changes in both systolic and diastolic blood pressures. In general, side-effects were of limited severity and included tiredness (which was circumvented by giving the tablets at night) and impotence ($n = 3$). Twenty-five of the original 48 remained on treatment for over 2 years.

Lepor *et al.* (1991) have summarized the non-randomized data-base for treatment of symptomatic BPH with terazosin. A total of 163 men were entered in four separate clinical trials. Dosage ranged from 5 mg to 20 mg. Results showed overall improvement in peak and mean flow rates of 41% and 43% while symptom scores showed a decrease of 62% for obstructive symptoms and of 33% for irritative symptoms. Changes in systolic and diastolic blood pressure were minimal.

The safety and efficacy of terazosin were recently evaluated in a randomized placebo-controlled multi-centre trial Lepor *et al.* (1992). Three hundred and fourteen men were entered and randomly allocated to placebo, 2, 5 or 10 mg of terazosin. All treatment groups exhibited symptomatic improvement compared with the placebo group, while the 10 mg terazosin group showed statistically increased peak and mean flow rates compared with the placebo group. The incidence of side-effects was not statistically increased in the treated group. This large study demonstrates the efficacy and safety of 10 mg of terazosin.

Alpha-reductase inhibitors

Compounds which inhibit the enzyme 5-alpha-reductase prevent conversion of testosterone to dihydrotestosterone (DHT). The concept of using 5-alpha-reductase inhibitors in the treatment of BPH arose from a unique study of a rare autosomal recessive gene-mediated metabolic disorder known as congenital 5-alpha-reductase deficiency. At birth, these genotypic males (karyotype 46 XY) with congenital 5-alpha-reductase deficiency presented with ambiguous genitalia. They had, however, normal male internal duct structures and normally differentiated testes. The patients described by Imperato-McGinley *et al.* (1974) all came from a single village in the Dominican Republic. These boys were initially raised as girls till puberty, when testosterone levels increased and they developed normal-sized penises and deep voices. However, postpubertal examination showed that they had very small prostates, scanty beard and no acne or temple hair recession with normal libido.

These changes occur as urogenital sinus-derived structures such as the prostate require DHT for growth, while Wolffian duct-derived structures such as the epididymis and vas deferens which depend on testosterone for growth are normal as testosterone production is unaffected in this condition. The synthetic compound finasteride (MK-906, Proscar) is a 4-aza-steroid compound which has potent *in vivo* 5-alpha-reductase-inhibitory action, but does not appear to interfere with testosterone or binding of DHT to its receptor. It also has no androgenic or anti-androgenic characteristics or any other recognizable hormonal properties. Thus, the very selective nature of this group of compounds which reduce DHT levels without other hormonal effects appear beneficial in the treatment of BPH.

The influence of finasteride on the volume of the peripheral and periurethral zones of the prostate in men with BPH

A large randomized placebo-controlled phase III clinical trial in North America (Stoner, 1991), using finasteride 5 mg once daily for one year to treat symptomatic BPH, reported decrease in prostate volume by 20%, increase in mean urinary peak flow by 1.5 ml/s and reduction in total symptom scores (obstructive and irritative) by 1.5 points approximately. Finasteride reduced plasma DHT by 70% with a 10% increase in serum testosterone. A nearly 50% decrease in PSA (prostatic specific antigen) levels was also noted. Side-effects were minimal. The only significant side-effect appeared to be impotence (3.7% in treatment group compared with 1.1% for controls).

A recent study from Johns Hopkins has demonstrated reduction in size of the periurethral zone of the prostate following alpha-reductase inhibitor. Tempany *et al.* (1993) randomized 20 symptomatic men with BPH to treatment with finasteride 1 mg/day, finasteride 5 mg/day and placebo. Prostate volume was measured by 3-D reconstructions of magnetic resonance contoured images of the prostate. After 1 year's therapy with finasteride there was no significant difference in the two treatment arms. A statistically significant decrease in the size of the periurethral lobe was noted in the treatment group compared with placebo (6.2 ± 3 ml) ($P < 0.03$). There was also a significant decrease in total gland size and a non-significant decrease in size of the peripheral zone. This study demonstrated for the first time a significant reduction following 5-alpha reductase inhibitor therapy of the periurethral zone, which is the region responsible for urethral obstruction.

Finasteride

A recent study from Johns Hopkins has demonstrated reduction in size of the periurethral zone of the prostate following 5-reductase therapy. Tempany *et al.* (1993) randomized 20 symptomatic men with BPH to treatment with finasteride 1 mg/day, finasteride 5 mg/day and placebo. Prostate volume was measured by 3-D reconstructions of magnetic resonance contoured images of the prostate. After 1 year's therapy with finasteride there was no significant difference in the two treatments. A statistically significant decrease in the size of the periurethral lobe was noted in the treatment group compared with placebo (6.2 + 3 ml) ($P < 0.03$). There was also a significant decrease in total gland size and a non-significant decrease in size of the peripheral zone.

This study demonstrated for the first time a significant reduction, following 5-reductase therapy, of the periurethral zone which is the region responsible for urethral obstruction.

Androgen suppression and aromatase inhibitors

The basic rationale for androgen suppression in the clinical treatment of BPH arises from the knowledge that androgens are essential for prostate growth. It is well known that BPH does not occur in men who have been castrated before puberty and rarely if orchidectomy has taken place before the age of 40. It has also been observed that regression of established BPH can occur with anti-androgen treatment. White (1985) reported that 87% of 111 patients with BPH treated by bilateral orchidectomy had significant reduction of prostate size as judged by digital rectal examination. Cabot (1986) reported similar results in 61 men and found that 84% noted improved ability to void after orchidectomy.

Laboratory tests have shown that BPH can be reproduced in rats and dogs by androgen or a combination of androgen and oestrogenic stimulation. Ehrlichman *et al.* (1981) produced significant prostatic enlargement in castrated rats with atrophied prostates by administering DHT or DHT plus 17-β-oestradiol. In a similar experiment Walsh and Wilson (1976) induced glandular BPH in castrated beagles by the combined treatment with 17-β-oestradiol and 3-alpha-androstanediol. Following this other researchers were able to demonstrate prostatic hyperplasia in previously castrated dogs by administering concomitantly DHT and 17-β-oestradiol. These experiments show that testicular androgens are important in the pathogenesis of BPH.

Physiology of androgen production

The testes produce more than 90% of the total androgen. The remaining 5–10% comes from the adrenals as products of sterol biosynthetics. Testicular androgen production is under the control of the hypothalamus–pituitary axis. Nerve cells in the pre-optic hypothalamus secrete the decapeptide gonadotrophin-releasing hormone (GnRH). This release of GnRH occurs in a pulsatile fashion directly from the nerve terminals into the hypophyseal portal circulation. GnRH then binds to high-affinity receptors on the cell membrane of anterior pituitary cells. The anterior pituitary cells are thus stimulated to produce the heterodimeric gonadotrophins, follicle-stimulating hormone (FSH) and luteinizing hormone (LH).

The LH released into the peripheral circulation reaches the testes and binds to specific receptors on Leydig cells present in the testes. The Leydig cells are thus stimulated to produce testosterone primarily. This testosterone travels in the blood stream in the free state and is also bound to specific sex hormone-binding globulin (SHBG) and albumin. At the target organ (the prostate), free testosterone binds to receptors on the surface of the prostatic cell. The majority is converted to DHT. This conversion takes place under the influence of the enzyme 5-alpha-reductase. The remaining testosterone and DHT then bind to specific high-affinity androgen receptor protein and enter the nucleus by the process of transformation and translocation. Inside the nucleus, the androgen–receptor complex interacts with specific DNA binding sites. Androgen-dependent genes undergo transcription which results in production of messenger RNA (mRNA). Synthesis of specific proteins and enzymes are produced by the process of translation. Overall, there is a net increase in protein biosynthesis resulting in cellular hypertrophy and hyperplasia. Thus, blocks at various levels in this chain have an effect on prostatic cell growth.

Aromatase inhibitors

It is well known that the pathogenesis of BPH is under hormonal control and it is believed that oestrogens and androgens act synergistically to control prostatic growth. In fact, high concentrations of oestrogen receptors are present in the prostatic stroma which is the predominant tissue element in BPH. In man, oestrogen production takes place mainly by the peripheral aromatization of testicular and adrenal androgens. Therefore, aromatase inhibitors which inhibit the biosynthesis of oestrogen in the male have been investigated as prospective therapeutic modulators of BPH. Initial studies have been carried out on animal models.

Scientific basis of research in aromatase inhibitors

In males, the oestrogenic substances oestrone and 17-β-oestradiol are produced exclusively by aromatization of androstenedione and testosterone. This chemical conversion is performed by the microsomal cytochrome P-450-dependent enzyme system, otherwise commonly known as aromatase, which has a molecular weight of 55 000 daltons.

The first aromatase inhibitor to be used in the treatment of BPH was 4-hydroxyandrostenedione (4-OHA). Habenicht *et al.* (1986) studied 14 beagles and examined the effects of androstenedione and 4-OHA on the prostate after orchidectomy. They found that treatment with androstendione resulted in BPH exclusively characterized by oestrogenic effects such as growth of smooth muscle and cystic enlargement of acini and ducts which suggest stromal stimulation. This oestrogen-related stromal growth could be inhibited by subsequent treatment with 4-OHA. The epithelial hyperplastic effects were also partially antagonized by 4-OHA.

In a further study, Habenicht and El Etreby (1987) investigated the possibility of antagonizing androstenedione-induced stromal changes in the prostates of castrated dogs by treatment with an aromatase inhibitor and also whether it was possible to produce a synergistic effect by adding the anti-androgen cyproterone acetate to the aromatase inhibitor. The aromatase inhibitor used in this study, 1-methyl-ADD, completely antagonized all the oestrogen-induced changes in the prostates of these castrated dogs.

By adding cyproterone acetate (CPA) there was an additional synergistic inhibitory effect on both the epithelial and stromal compounds of the prostate. Histological sections showed that the appearances of the prostate treated with both aromatase inhibitors and anti-androgen was similar to that of untreated castrate controls. Thus this study indicates that a combination of anti-oestrogens and anti-androgens may be the one that produces the best overall results in BPH treatment.

In a third study, Habenicht and El Etreby (1989) studied the effect of combined CPA and 1-methyl-ADD therapy for prostatic growth induced by androstendione in intact beagles. 1-Methyl-ADD antagonized the oestrogen-induced growth in the fibromuscular stromal element; however, it also produced a marked counter-regularity increase in serum testosterone and DHT levels which led to marked hyperplasia of the glandular element of the prostate. This pronounced rise in serum testosterone and DHT is due to absence of negative feedback by oestrogens at the hypothalamic and pituitary levels. Lack of oestrogens prevents the inhibitory regulation of the hypothalamus and pituitaty which leads to excess LH production which in turn leads to increased testicular testosterone production with subsequent conversion to DHT. The effect of this androgenic surge on the prostate can, however, be completely blocked by CPA. Thus when CPA and 1-methyl-ADD were used in combination there was complete atrophy of the prostate despite a sharp elevation of the serum testosterone and DHT levels.

In a clinical study of 13 men with indwelling catheters treated with the weak aromatase inhibitor testolactone, seven were able to void spontaneously after 8 weeks of treatment. In these men, the prostate was noted to shrink by an average of 26% (Schweikert & Tunn, 1987). More potent compounds such as 1-methyl-ADD have as described above been shown to inhibit oestrogen-induced growth of the prostatic stroma in animals. However, no clinical data corroborating their efficacy in man have been published.

Luteinizing-hormone-releasing-hormone (LHRH) agonists

LHRH analogues have a protein structure which is very similar to naturally occurring human LHRH. They bind with great affinity to the LHRH receptor on the cell membrane of the gonadotrophic cells of the anterior pituitary. These analogues have a considerably greater ability to bind to the LHRH receptor and are more resistant to proteolytic degradation. When LHRH agonists are continuously administered, i.e. in a non-pulsatile manner, there is down-regulation or desensitization of the LHRH–receptor complex on the surface of the cells of the anterior pituitary. This leads to decreased stimulation of the cells and decreased gonadotrophin synthesis. Eventually, after several weeks of continuous therapy, FSH and LH cease to be secreted. This results in absence of stimulation of the Leydig cells of the testes leading to stoppage of testicular androgen production. Testosterone drops to castrate levels ($< 50\,\mu g/dl$).

The androgen which remains in the blood stream is derived from the adrenal glands and accounts for 5–10% of normal total androgen production. Thus only a minimal amount of testosterone enters the prostate cell. The critical level of androgen required to maintain the hyperplastic state of BPH is not reached, and involution of stromal hyperplasia occurs.

Animal models were used to study LHRH agonists in the early 1980s. Since then a number of clinical trials have been reported. Peters and Walsh (1987) used the GnRH agonist Nafaselin acetate 400 mg daily in nine men with proven bladder outflow obstruction due to BPH. The trial lasted 6 months. Serum testosterone was reduced to castrate levels and the prostate size decreased by 24.2% on average. Six men had symptomatic improvement, but only half of them had improved flow rates. All were rendered impotent and experienced hot flushes. Serum testosterone levels and prostatic volumes returned to pre-treatment levels 6 months after cessation of treatment.

Gabrilove *et al.* (1989) used leuprolide in 15 men with BPH. Prostatic size reduced by 40% on average after 4 months and 46% after 6 months. Flow rates and obstructive symptoms improved in all with some improvements in irritative symptoms. Of five with indwelling catheters, three were able to void spontaneously after treatment. Impotence and hot flushes occurred in all the men.

Natural plant extracts (phytotherapy)

Plant extracts are widely used in some countries, especially Germany, for the symptomatic treatment of BPH. This is known as phytotherapy. Common plant sources include the seed of the pumpkin, *Cucurbita pepo*, and the fruit of the dwarf palm, *Sabal serrulatum*.

It has been suggested that the active ingredients of these plant extracts are related to steroids such as sitosterols and phytosterols. Suggested mechanisms of action include reduction of plasma cholesterol levels, inhibition of testosterone binding to androgen receptors and inhibition of DHT production. Although some *in vitro* effects have been demonstrated, *in vivo* effects remain uncertain.

Review of the literature shows conflicting results with only four good placebo-controlled trials (Dreikorn & Richter, 1989). Improvements in flow rate and symptomatology have been reported with *Cucurbita pepo* and *Sabal serrulatum*, while a pollen extract from Cernilton®, Switzerland has been claimed to decrease prostate size (Buck *et al.*, 1990). In spite of these reports, there is little evidence to support the view that phytotherapy has any significant benefit over placebo. Perhaps it is for this reason that the discerning urological community in the United Kingdom has been hitherto resistant to the wider use of plant extracts to treat BPH.

Overview

At the time of writing, of all the medical agents available, alpha-blockers and the 5-alpha-reductase inhibitor, finasteride, are the ones in common use in the United Kingdom. Phytotherapy although popular in the continent is not used widely in this country.

As we have seen, there is good scientific evidence for the use of alpha-blockers while 5-alpha-reductase inhibitors have been proven to shrink the prostate. In theory, the idea of a combination of alpha-blockers to relax the prostatic musculature and 5-alpha-reductase inhibitors to reduce the volume of the adenoma would appear attractive. Good-quality controlled clinical trials would prove the efficacy or otherwise of this concept. Certainly the search for newer more prostate-specific alpha-blockers continues and recent studies have demonstrated sub-types of alpha-1-adrenoceptor: alpha-1A, alpha-1B and alpha-1C, of which the last, i.e. alpha-1C, seems to form the majority in the prostatic population (Chapple *et al.*, 1991; Marshall *et al.*, 1992).

At present, the use of medical treatment is restricted to those men who are not in imminent danger from the more serious effects of BPH. Therefore, patients with impaired renal function due to bladder outlet obstruction, recurrent urinary tract infection (UTI), acute or chronic retention and those with bladder stones are not suitable for drug therapy. Medical treatment should be considered for those who have mild symptoms and in whom dangerous sequelae as enumerated above have been excluded. Men on waiting lists for prostatectomy may also be offered medical treatment, as well as those who refuse surgery.

References

Abrams P.H., Shah P.J.R., Stone A.R. & Choa R.G. (1982) Bladder outflow obstruction treated with phenoxybenzamine. *Br. J. Urol.*, **54**, 527–30.

Bartsch G., Muller H.R., Oberholzer M. & Rohr H.P. (1979) Light microscopic stereological analysis of the normal human prostate and of benign prostatic hyperplasia. *J. Urol.*, **122**, 487–91.

Boreham P.F., Braithwaite P., Milewski P. & Pearson H. (1977) Alpha-adrenergic blockers in prostatism. *Br. J. Surg.*, **64**, 756–7.

Brooks M.E., Sidi A.A., Hanani Y. & Braf Z.F. (1983) Ineffectiveness of phenoxybenzamine in treatment of benign prostatic hypertrophy. A controlled study. *Urology*, **21**, 474–8.

Buck A.C., Cox R., Rees R.W., Ebeling J. & John A. (1990) Treatment of outflow tract obstruction due to benign prostatic hyperplasia with the pollen extract, Cernilton. *Br. J. Urol.*, **66**, 398–404.

Cabot A.T. (1986) The question of castration for enlarged prostate. *Ann. Surg.*, **24**, 265–309.

Caine M., Raz S. & Zeigler M. (1975) Adrenergic and cholinergic receptors in the human prostate, prostatic capsule and bladder neck. *Br. J. Urol.*, **47**, 193–202.

Caine M., Perlberg S. & Meretyk S. (1978) A placebo-controlled double-blind study of the effect of phenoxybenzamine in benign prostatic obstruction. *Br. J. Urol.*, **50**, 551–4.

Chapple C.R., Aubry M.L., James S. *et al.* (1989) Characterisation of human prostatic adrenoceptors using pharmacology receptor binding and localisation. *Br. J. Urol.*, **63**, 487–96.

Chapple C.R., Burt R. & Marshall I. (1991) Adrenoceptor subtypes in the human prostate and inferior epigastric artery. *Neurourol. Urodyn.*, **10**, 306–8.

Chow W., Hahn D., Sandhu D. *et al.*, (1990) Multicentre controlled trial of Indoramin in the symptomatic relief of benign prostatic hypertrophy. *Br. J. Urol.*, **65**, 36–8.

Dreikorn K. & Richter R. (1989) Conservative nonhormonal treatment of patients with benign prostatic hyperplasia. In: Ackermann R. & Schroder F.H. (eds) Prostatic Hyperplasia. Etiology, Surgical and Conservative Management, pp. 109–121. De Gruyter, Berlin.

Ehrlichman R.J., Isaacs J.T. & Coffey D.S. (1981) Differences in the effects of estradiol on dihydrotestosterone induced prostatic growth of the castrate dog and rat. *Invest. Urol.*, **18**, 466–70.

Ferrie B.G. & Paterson P.J. (1986) Phenoxybenzamine in prostatic hypertrophy. *Br. J. Urol.*, **59**, 63–5.

Gabrilove J.L., Levine A.C., Kirschenbaum A. & Droller M. (1989) Effect of long-acting gonadotropin-releasing hormone analog (leuprolide) therapy on prostatic size and symptoms in 15 men with benign prostatic hypertrophy. *J. Clin. Endocrinol. Metab.*, **69**, 629–32.

Habenicht U.-F. & El Etreby M.F. (1987) Synergic inhibitory effects of the aromatase inhibitor 1-methyl-androsta-1, 4-diene-3, 17-dione and the antiandrogen cyproterone acetate on androstenedione-induced hyperplastic effects in the prostates of castrated dogs. *Prostate*, **11**, 133–43.

Habenicht U.-F. & El Etreby M.F. (1989) Selective inhibition of androstenedione-induced prostate growth in intact beagle dogs by a combined treatment with the antiandrogen cyproterone acetate and the aromatase inhibitor 1-methyl-androsta-1, 4-diene-3, 17-dione (1-methyl-ADD). *Prostate*, **14**, 309–22.

Habenicht U.-F., Schwartz K., Schweikert H.U., Neumann F. & El Etreby M.F. (1986) Development of a model for the induction of estrogen-related prostatic hyperplasia in the dog and its response to the aromatase inhibitor 4-hydroxy-4-androstene-3, 17-dione: preliminary results. *Prostate*, **8**, 181–94.

Hedlund H., Andersson K.E. & Ek A. (1983) Effects of prazosin in patients with benign prostatic obstruction. *J. Urol.*, **130**, 275–8.

Iacovou J.W. & Dunn M. (1987) Indoramin — an effective new drug in the management of bladder outflow obstruction. *Br. J. Urol.*, **60**, 526–8.

Imperato-McGinley J., Guerrero L., Gautier T. & Peterson R.E. (1974) Steroid 5α-reductase deficiency in man: an inherited form of male pseudohermaphroditism. *Science*, **186**, 1213–15.

Kirby R.S., Coppinger S.W.C., Corcoran M.O., Chapple C.R., Flannagan M. & Milroy E.J.G. (1987) Prazosin in the treatment of prostatic obstruction. A placebo-controlled study. *Br. J. Urol.*, **60**, 136–42.

Lepor H., Knapp-Maloney G. & Sunshine H. (1990) A dose titration study evaluating terazosin, a selective, once-a-day α_1-blocker for the treatment of symptomatic benign prostatic hyperplasia. *J. Urol.*, **144**, 1393–98.

Lepor H., Henry D. & Ladddu A.R. (1991) The efficacy and safety of terazosin for the treatment of symptomatic BPH. *Prostate*, **18**, 345–55.

Lepor H., Auerbach S., Puras-Baez A. *et al.* (1992) A randomized, placebo-controlled multicenter study of the efficacy and safety of terazosin in the treatment of benign prostatic hyperplasia. *J. Urol.*, **148**, 1467–74.

Marshall I., Burt R., Andersson P.O., Chapple C.R., Greengrass P.M., Johnson G.I. & Wyllie M.G. (1992) Human adrenoceptor: functional characterisation in prostate. *Br. J. Pharmacol.*, **107** (Proc. Suppl.), 327P.

Martorana G., Giberti C., Damonte P. *et al.* (1984) The effect of prazosin in benign prostatic hypertrophy: A placebo-controlled double-blind study. *IRCS Med. Sci.*, **12**, 11–12.

Peters C.A. & Walsh P.C. (1987) The effect of Nafarelin acetate, a luteinizing hormone-releasing hormone agonist, on benign prostatic hyperplasia. *N. Engl. J. Med.*, **317**, 599–604.

Schweikert H.-U. & Tunn U.W. (1987) Effects of the aromatase inhibitor testolactone on human benign prostatic hyperplasia. *Steroids*, **50**, 191–200.

Stoner E.J. (1991) Phase III studies evaluating 5α-reductase inhibitor, Proscar.

American Urological Association Annual Meeting, Toronto, Ontario, Canada. 2–6 June.

Stott M.A. & Abrams P.H. (1991) Indoramin in the treatment of prostatic bladder outflow obstruction. *Br. J. Urol.*, **67**, 499–501.

Tempany C.M., Partin A.W., Zerhouni E.A., Zinreich S.J. & Walsh P.C. (1993) The influence of Finasteride on the volume of the peripheral and periurethral zones of the prostate in men with benign prostatic hyperplasia. *The Prostate*, **22**, 39–42.

Thien T., Delaere K.P., Debruyne F.M. & Koene R.A.P. (1987) Urinary incontinence caused by prazosin. *Br. Med. J.*, **i**, 622–3.

Walsh P.C. & Wilson J.D. (1976) The induction of prostatic hypertrophy in the dog with androstanediol. *J. Clin. Invest.*, **57**, 1093–7.

White J.W. (1985) The results of double castration in hypertrophy of the prostate. *Ann. Surg.*, **22**, 1–80.

4 Ultrasound-guided techniques

C.R. CHARIG

Introduction

Transrectal ultrasound (TRUS) has greatly improved our understanding and hence management of prostatic and other urological conditions. However, what is not fully appreciated about this modality is the great versatility with which it can be used and the numerous applications in both diagnostic and therapeutic fields.

Although TRUS is not a new field of investigation (Watanabe *et al.*, 1980) and we owe a debt to British urologists for its development (Peeling & Griffiths, 1984), it is only in the last few years that any great interest has been expressed by urologists in the United Kingdom. This has come about primarily from improvement in the equipment and also from renewed interest in the management of carcinoma of the prostate. In an ideal world, TRUS should be available to all surgeons, and I hope in the course of this chapter to show many of the new-found applications of ultrasound.

I shall divide the practical aspects of TRUS into three main areas: diagnostic; therapeutic; and experimental (Table 4.1). Under each heading I shall discuss the main applications with some practical advice on how to perform certain procedures. Where these procedures are discussed more fully elsewhere in this book, I shall give a brief description of the technique, and present our results at St Peter's Hospital. For the purposes of this presentation I have had to assume that the reader has a basic understanding of ultrasound, and an ability to interpret the images. This can only come with practice and experience. It cannot be taught.

The main feature, which is common to all these techniques and why ultrasound is so important, is accuracy. Apart from affording the best means of visualizing the prostate gland and associated structures, TRUS allows accurate measurement of size, volume, and prostatic dimensions, as well as accurate location of lesions into which a needle can be introduced. The current therapeutic trend is towards minimal disturbance to the patient. Here too ultrasound has an important role in allowing treatments aimed solely at the gland itself, and visualizing the changes after using certain newer treatment modalities, i.e. heating, cooling, and irradiating.

Table 4.1. Three main areas of TRUS

Diagnostic	*Therapeutic*
Volumetric analysis	^{125}I seed implantation
Prostatic biopsy	Second-look TURP
— Transperineal	Laser 'prostatectomy'
— transrectal	Bladder-neck suspension
Aspiration cytology	Balloon dilatation
Seminal vesicle aspiration	Microwave hyperthermia
Dynamic vasography	
Combination urodynamics	*Experimental*
Stress incontinence	Interstitial laser hyperthermia
	Cryoprostatectomy
	Endoscopic liquidization
	Computer-aided TURP

Diagnostic procedures

Volumetric analysis

This is a very important aspect of ultrasound diagnosis when investigating outflow obstruction in the male (Watanabe *et al.*, 1974). Although there is little correlation between size and symptoms, volume estimation can give the answer in a lot of cases, usually as a negative finding, i.e. when glands are very small, they can usually be discounted as a cause of obstruction. Knowing the size of the gland preoperatively is helpful. Where a very large gland (Fig. 4.1) is found, a retropubic prostatectomy may save the ordeal of having to resect an 80–100 g prostate. In the assessment of post-operative voiding problems, an ultrasound estimation of prostate volume may show a large amount of residual prostate as the cause of continuing obstruction after surgery. In one recent series, an average of only 40% of the prostate gland was ever resected by most surgeons.

There are three techniques for measuring volume: the planimetric, ellipsoidal and two-plane methods.

Planimetric volume measurements This is considered to be the most accurate (± 10%) but is also the most time-consuming. It is computed by summating the areas for a number of slices along the length of the prostate. The gland is scanned in the axial plane, and the bladder neck and apex are identified as the limits of the prostatic urethra. The probe is mounted on a ratchet system that allows it to be moved in 5 mm gradations along the prostate (Fig. 4.2). The perimeter of each slice is drawn with a light pen, and the area and volume (V) are calculated by the software within the machine. This is repeated usually six to eight times in the average prostate. The calculation is given by

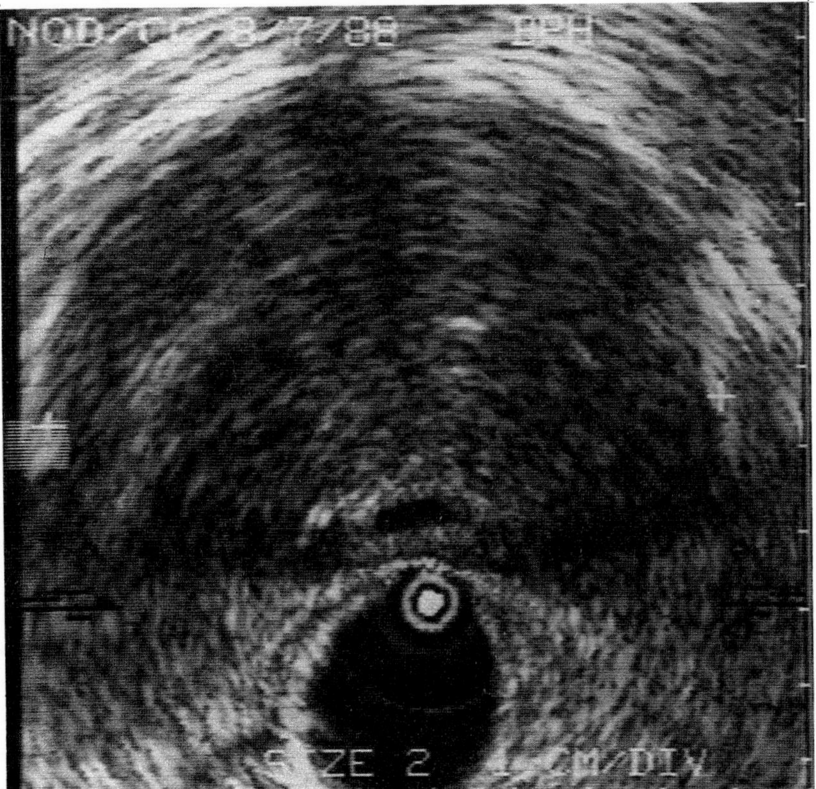

Fig. 4.1. Large BPH, 203 g, 8.7 × 6.5 × 5.5 cm.

$$V = \frac{L^2}{4\pi} \times T \times C$$

where L = perimeter, T = thickness of slice, and C = constant (approx 0.7).

Ellipsoidal method Whereas the first method calculates the volume based on a circle, with a correction factor, this method bases its computations on the prostate being ellipsoidal. This is not as accurate (± 20%), but is far quicker. The scanning technique is the same but the perimeter is only measured once, at the widest part of the gland, and the width of the gland is also recorded. The volume is then calculated from

$$V = \frac{8L^2}{3\pi D}$$

where L = the perimeter, and D = the maximum width of the gland.

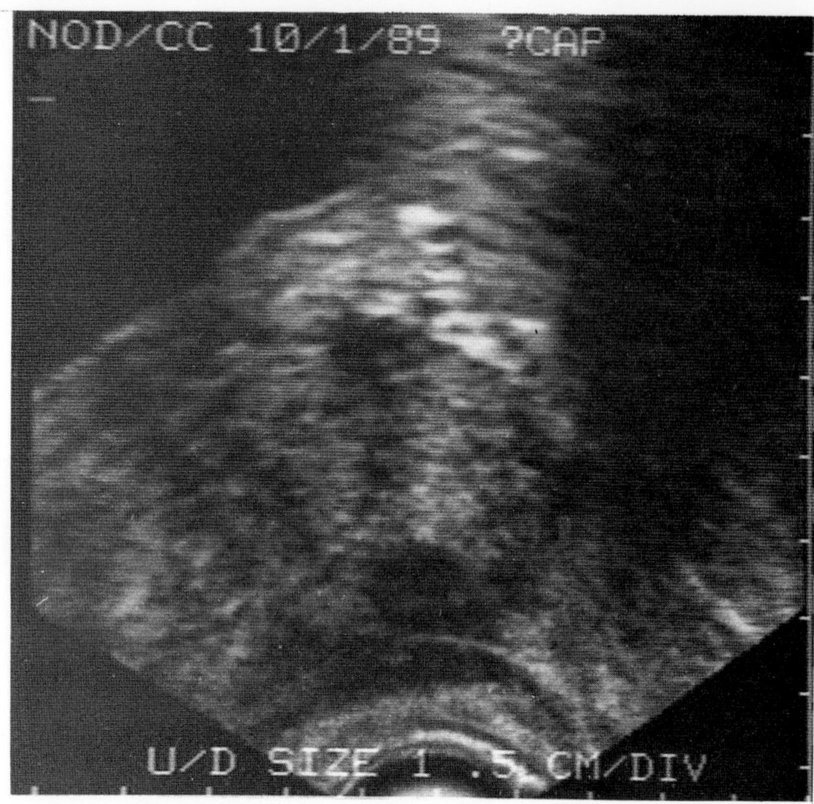

Fig. 4.2. Small tumour at apex, 0.8 × 0.7 cm.

Two-plane method This is the least accurate method and involves scanning in two planes. This is a cuboidal method and involves measuring three diameters: the A–P diameter and width on the axial view and the prostatic length on the sagittal view. The volume is derived from

$$V = D1 \times D2 \times D3 \times 0.7$$

where $D1$ = A–P diameter, $D2$ = width and $D3$ = length.

Prostatic biopsy

This can be carried out by two different routes: transperineal and transrectal. Both of these methods are accurate. Transrectal biopsy is easier for the patient but is often criticized by clinicians as being a potential route of infection. The real progress has come from careful histological examination and comparison with the images obtained on transrectal ultrasound. It is now accepted that tumours are hypoechoic in about 90% of cases (Lee *et al.*, 1985) but there are the exceptions of iso- or hyper-echoic tumours. However, we adopt a policy of biopsying any suspicious lesion. This does increase the number of negative biopsies, but we hope lessens the risk of missing a tumour.

Transperineal biopsy This is usually carried out as a day-case procedure, with the use of local anesthetic and sedoanalgesia (Abe *et al.*, 1987). The patient is scanned in the lithotomy position and the perineum and prostatic capsule are infiltrated with 2% lignocaine. If the patient is very anxious, Medazolam is given intravenously. A 22 G spinal needle (100 mm) is the best for injecting the local. The perineal guide is attached to the probe, and the 'Biopty' needle and gun are used to remove a core of tissue (Fig. 4.3). The needles tend to blunt easily on the skin, and hence multiple biopsies can prove difficult with this method. Although I have not made a formal study, I feel that this method is more accurate for apical lesions as it can be difficult to angle up the transrectal probe acutely to sample the apex of the gland (Lee *et al.*, 1987). There have been a few reported cases of perineal seeding of tumour using this method.

Transrectal biopsy This is performed as an outpatient procedure, without the need for any anaesthetic. I tend to give the patients one dose of intravenous gentamicin 80 mg as prophylaxis and a 5-day course of

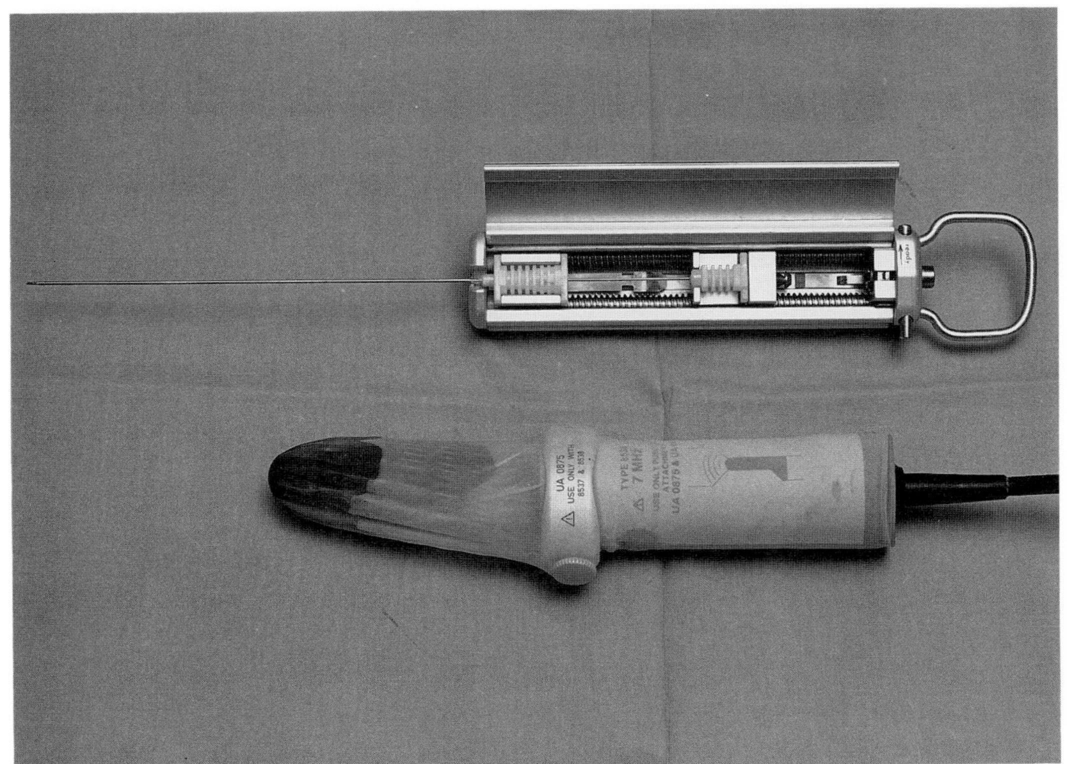

Fig. 4.3. Rectal probe with 'Biopty' gun and guide.

trimethoprim, and there have been no reported cases of UTI or bacteraemia to date. With the patient in either lithotomy or the left lateral position, and scanning in the sagittal plane, the probe plus needle guide is introduced into the rectum. An 18 G Biopty needle is advanced into the prostate until the needle is visible on the screen. The needle is then withdrawn 2 cm and the biopsy is taken with the aid of the Biopty gun, which fires the needle in one action. The scanning is done in the sagittal plane to ensure the correct depth of penetration into the gland, but the more modern probes allow one to scan in both the axial and the sagittal planes simultaneously, ensuring even greater accuracy of needle placement.

The 18 G Biopty needle and gun give a very adequate core of tissue for histological examination (Ragbe *et al.*, 1988). Multiple biopsies can be carried out without causing too much trauma either to the gland or to the patient. The patient should be warned to expect a certain amount of haematuria, lasting no longer than 24 hours. I have carried out over 150 biopsies using this technique, and have had no serious complications to date.

Aspiration cytology

If you are fortunate enough to work in a hospital with a good cytologist, then ultrasound-guided aspiration cytology is an extremely good diagnostic procedure. With the increasing use of flow cytometry as an investigative tool, small sample loads of as little as 10 000 cells can be analysed (Ronstrom *et al.*, 1981). The approaches to the prostate are the same as for a biopsy, except for cyst aspiration, where the transperineal route should be chosen to avoid the risk of turning the cyst into an abscess (Fig. 4.4). The aspirate is taken with the Lee-Ray 22 G needle, which has a side-on port and we have found this to be the best at the present time. Using this technique, one can also aspirate the seminal vesicles.

Dynamic vasography

This is an extremely good way to visualize the seminal vesicles (SVs) and to see whether the ejaculatory ducts are patent in the investigation of infertility. The vas deferens is exposed and cannulated in the scrotum, as for conventional vasography, and a weak solution of X-ray contrast and saline is injected antegradely through the vas. The fluid can be seen to pass through the SVs, through the ejaculatory ducts, into the prostatic urethra and thence to the bladder. Quite a large volume of fluid needs to be injected to overcome the dilatation of the SVs, especially when they are enlarged and atonic. This technique has shown up SVs which were not seen on X-ray and is also useful when trying to uncap or incise the ejaculatory ducts transurethrally (Fig. 4.5).

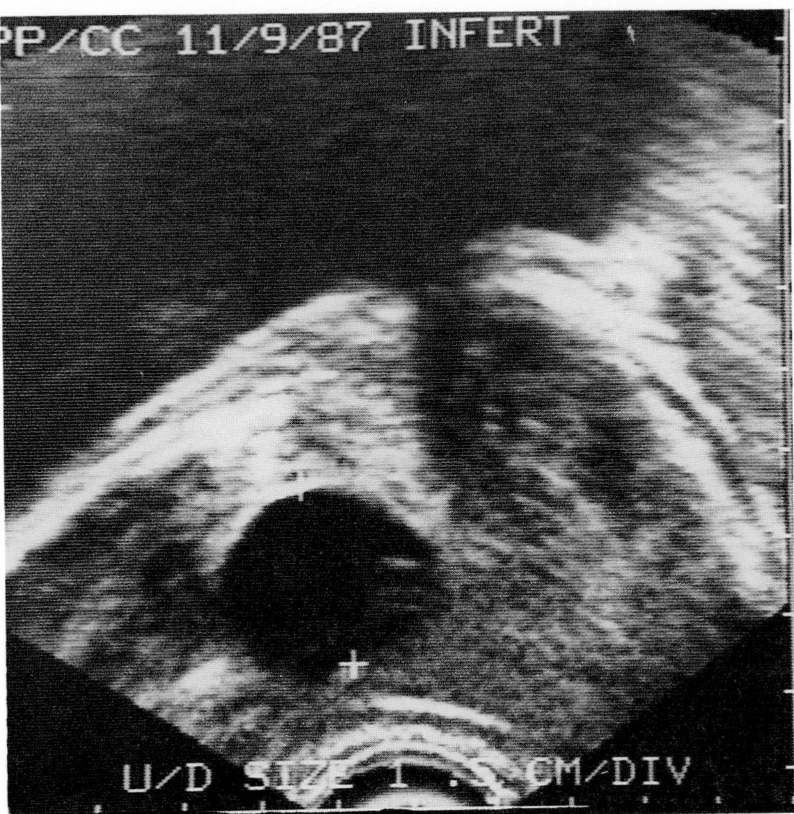

Fig. 4.4. Large cyst, 1.2 × 1.2 cm.

Combination TRUS and urodynamics

This is an interesting combination of investigative procedures, and is used mostly in spinal injury patients, where the need for X-rays in videocystometry has been replaced by ultrasound visualization of the bladder, bladder neck, and upper tracts (Shabesigh *et al.*, 1988). This enables the whole investigation to be carried out at the bedside and saves moving the patient to the X-ray department. The techniques are not difficult to combine and can be further refined to include urethral pressure profilometry and studies of the sphincter mechanisms when looking at incontinence.

Therapeutic

Interstitial ^{125}I seed implantation

One of the major benefits of transrectal ultrasound is that it opens up new therapeutic opportunities for a minimally invasive approach. This is of increasing importance when dealing with a disease such as prostate cancer, with such a varied natural history. The use of inter-

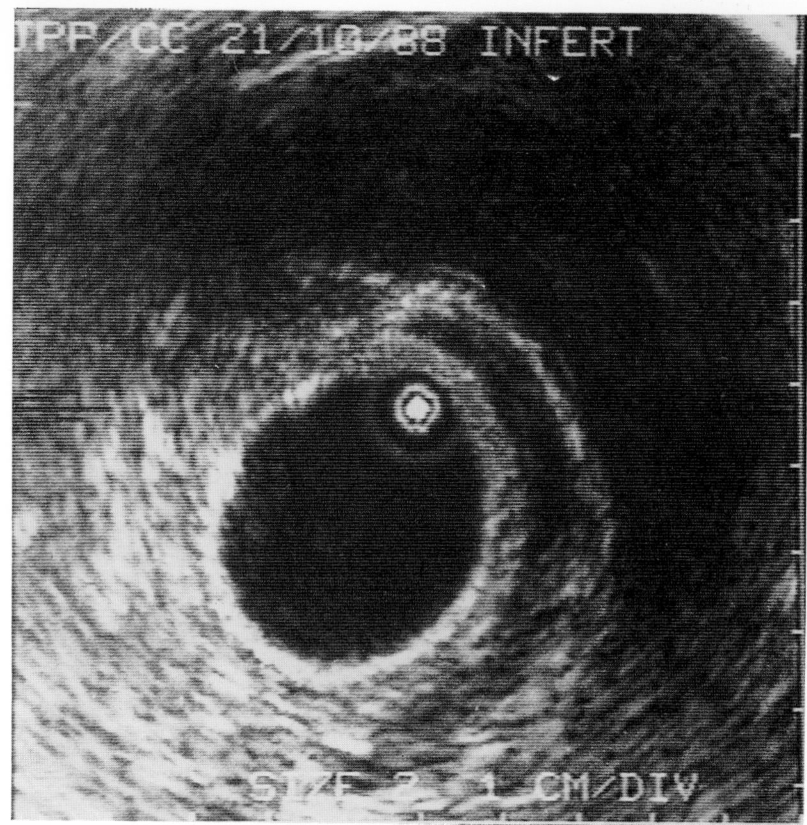

Fig. 4.5. Absent (right) seminal vesicle.

stitial radiation is not a new concept (Whitmore, 1980) but, with ultrasound, it is now possible to place the seeds transcutaneously, thereby removing the need for general anaesthetic. This reduces hospital stay to a matter of a couple of days (Fig. 4.6).

The technique is that developed by Holm and Stroyer in Copenhagen (Holm *et al.*, 1983). There is a planning stage, where the volume of the gland is measured. The matched peripheral dose, giving 160 Gy radiation, is then calculated by a physicist and the correct number of radioactive iodine needles are provided. A grid is attached to the ultrasound probe, which corresponds to a grid on the screen, when scanning in the axial plane. Long spinal needles (100) are then inserted through the grid-holes, which are 5 mm apart, through the perineal skin, and into the prostate gland, until they are seen on the screen to correspond to the matrix marks. The iodine seeds are then fed down the needles with buffers to separate them. In this way, 30–40 seeds can be introduced into the prostate.

We were part of a multi-centre trial but have now abandoned the technique after very poor results. Of the nine patients we treated by this method, two have died and four have progressive disease. The

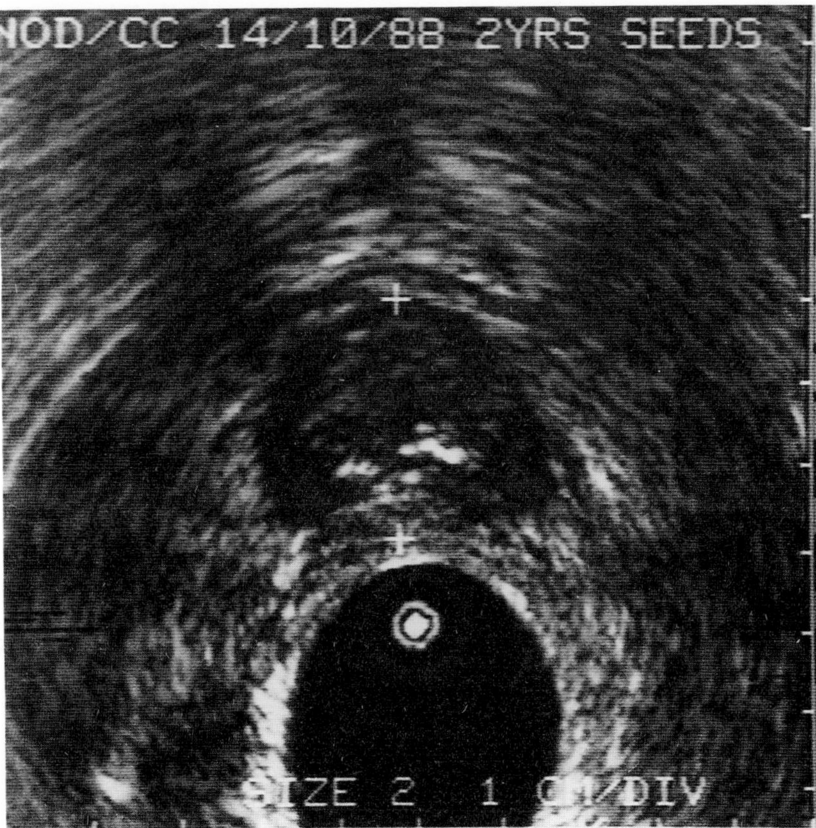

Fig. 4.6. Iodine seeds in prostate.

problem was one of under-dosing, which was a combination of poor planning, weak radioactive materials and the difficulty in placing the required number of needles in small-volume prostates. Our post-operative X-rays tended to show that the seeds had migrated into the bladder and surrounding tissues (Fig. 4.7). However, it should be stated that other groups have used this method very successfully (Cardiff, Oxford) and that the procedure itself is very well tolerated by patients.

Second-look transurethral resection of the prostate (TURP) for carcinoma of the prostate

This is a technique used in conjunction with Nd-YAG laser coagulation of the prostate, first described by Beisland & Sander (1986). The idea is to de-bulk the prostate as much as possible with the hot loop without endangering vital structures or perforating the capsule. With the ultrasound probe placed in the rectum during resection, the loop can be followed at all times and the depth of prostatic tissue remaining

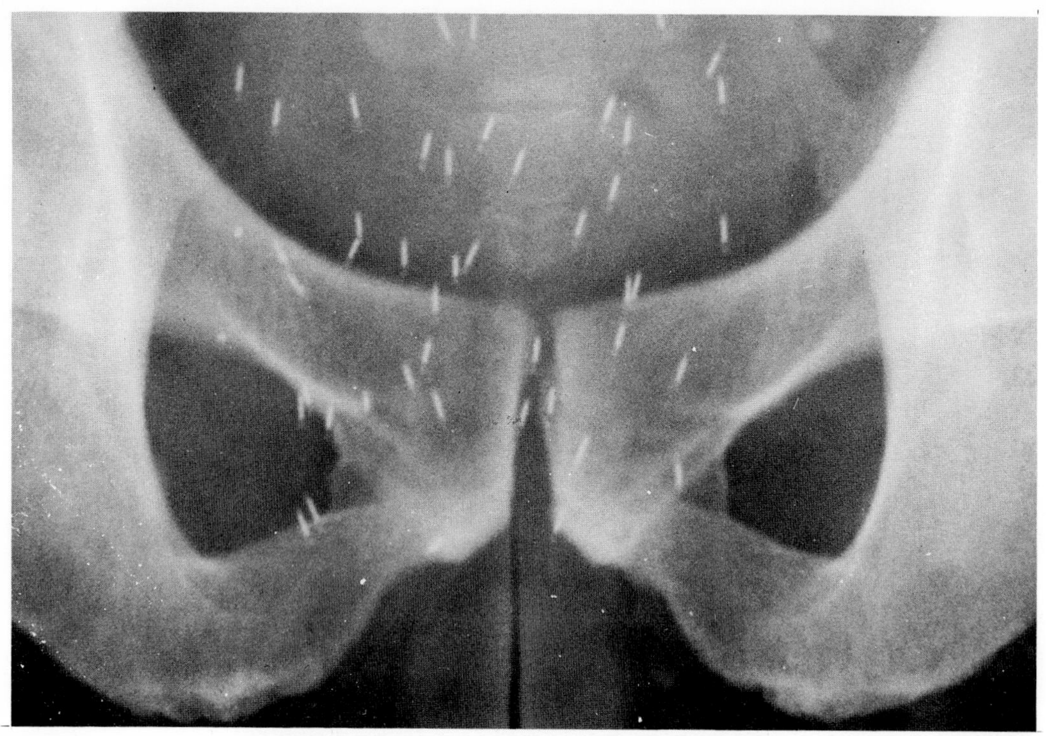

Fig. 4.7. X-ray of seeds in pelvis.

can be measured and the sphincter protected. A depth of less than 1 cm is aimed for throughout the prostate. The resection is carried out in quadrantic fashion around the clock-face for histological analysis. This may be a definitive form of treatment in its own right, or as a prelude to laser hyperthermia (Fig. 4.8).

Laser 'prostatectomy'

Following the second-look TURP, if there is further tumour in the specimen, the remaining capsule can be coagulated with the Nd-YAG laser. Pensel *et al.* (1981) have worked out that a power dose of 200 J (50 W for 4 s) causes thermal necrosis to a depth of 6 mm, and that the energy is far more controlled than with diathermy. The prostate is allowed to heal for 8–10 weeks, after the second-look TURP, and the gland is measured on ultrasound to ensure a depth of gland of less than 8–10 mm. A 600 μm quartz fibre is then passed down a modified resectoscope and the laser energy is applied to the remaining capsule. These patients are followed up very carefully with regular ultrasound and ultrasound-guided biopsies. We have treated 20 patients to date over the past 3 years, and there has been only one case of tumour progression (McNicholas *et al.*, 1988).

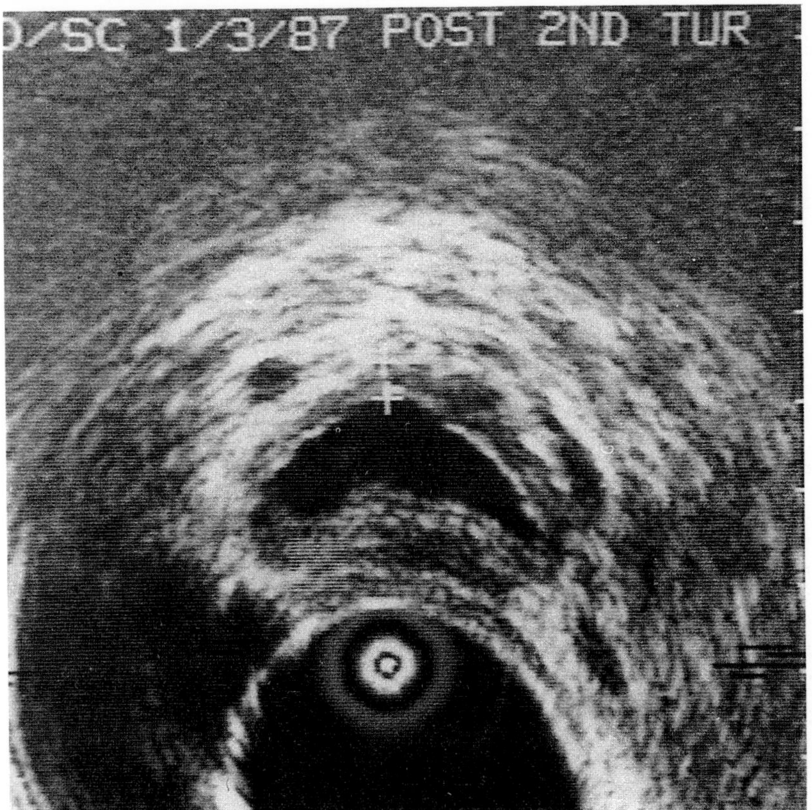

Fig. 4.8. Post second-look TURP.

Endoscopic bladder-neck suspension

We have been using the Bruel & Kjaer 8539 sagittal transducer transvaginally to treat women with stress incontinence. The probe can be used in the outpatient clinic to diagnose stress incontinence, providing excellent views of the bladder-neck opening and descent (Bergman *et al.*, 1988). Pre-operatively, the probe is placed in the vagina during the procedure of endoscopic bladder-neck suspension (Stamey or Pereyra-Raz) and left in the vagina once the tension sutures have been inserted (Fig. 4.9). These can then be tightened while the bladder neck is observed under ultrasound guidance. This technique can incorporate tension balancing, to ensure the right degree of bladder-neck elevation.

Balloon dilatation

This is a new form of treatment for BPH (Von Castenada *et al.*, 1987), currently being assessed in three centres in the United Kingdom. It involves the inflation of a 25–30 mm balloon at 5 atm in the

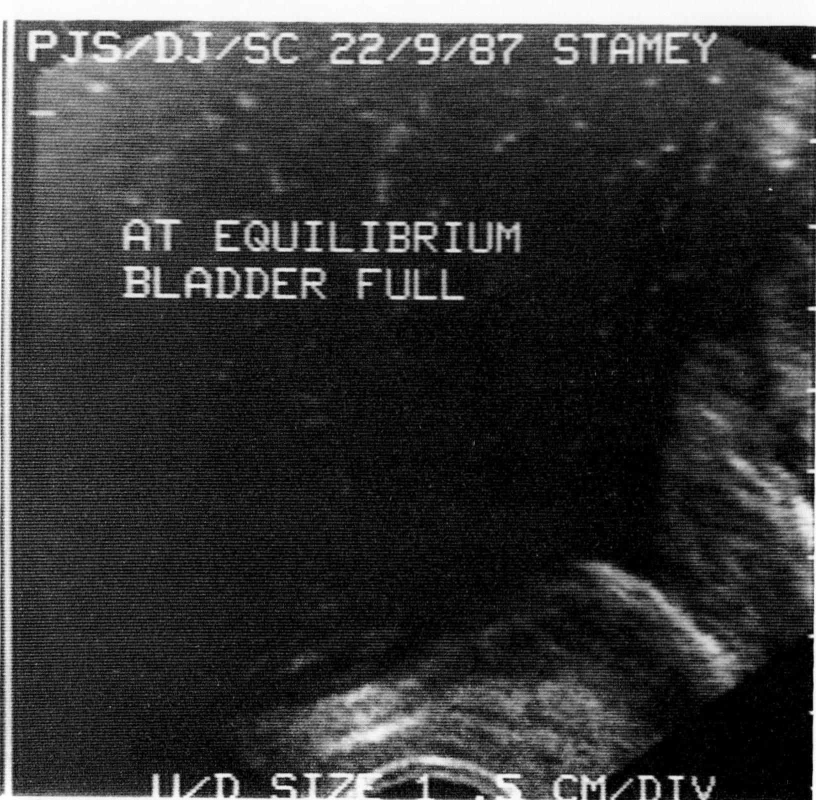

Fig. 4.9. Bladder neck during Stamey procedure.

prostatic urethra for approximately 10 minutes. This causes distraction of the lateral lobes and disruption of the bladder-neck fibres. The balloons can be inserted under direct vision, under fluoroscopy, or with ultrasound guidance. With ultrasound, the sphincters are easily identified, as is the balloon, and there is no harmful radiation. Our preliminary results with this procedure have been disappointing (Fig. 4.12, see also Chapter 5).

Microwave hyperthermia

This application of microwave technology, developed in Israel (Servadio *et al.*, 1987), allows heating of the prostate by an intrarectal probe or intrarectal pulse, in order to shrink the prostate in BPH. An integral part of the treatment involves monitoring the changes by ultrasound. Further information is presented in Chapter 8.

Potential new clinical uses

The following techniques all lend themselves extremely well to ultrasound imaging.

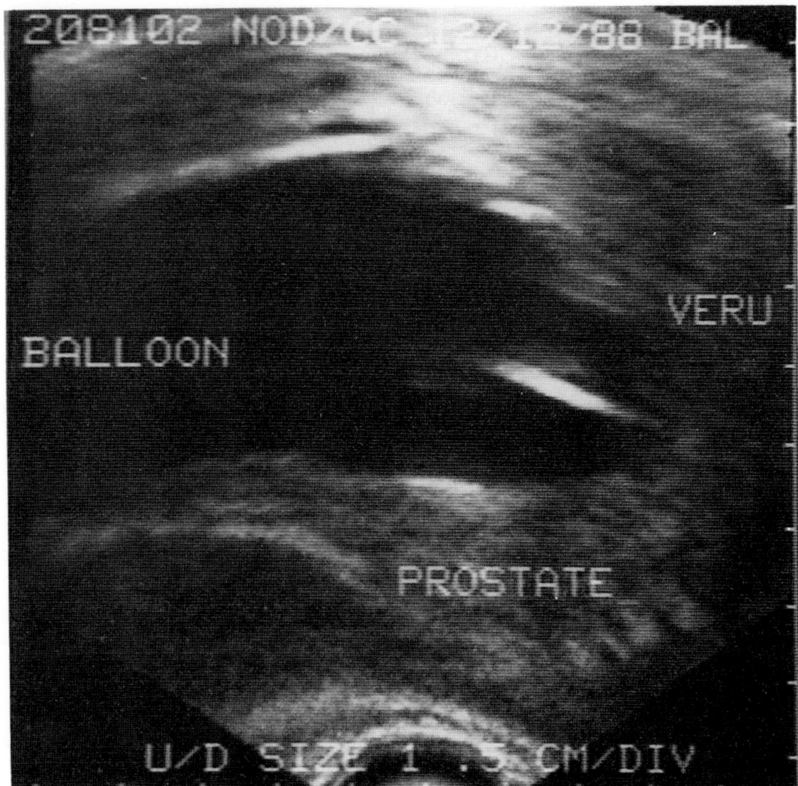

Fig. 4.10. Prostatotomy balloon inflated in prostate.

Interstitial laser hyperthermia

This is seen as an extrapolation of the laser 'prostatectomy'. Here a single fibre (or multiple fibres) is inserted directly into the prostate (into a small tumour or nodule) in an attempt to treat the tumours of very old or frail men, who might not tolerate an operation (Fig 4.10). There has been some encouraging animal work on the dosimetry which has clearly demonstrated that the small fibres and the areas of necrosis show up very well on ultrasound. This could provide a very accurate and atraumatic way of dealing with early cancers (Fig. 4.11).

Cryoprostatectomy

This has now fallen into disuse, although it was used extensively in Norwich, where the technique was pioneered (Green, 1970). Newer methods of cooling using nitrous oxide instead of liquid nitrogen have also been looked at, and the ice ball created in the prostate shows up remarkably well on ultrasound. The size of the ball can be measured, and its precise location can be monitored.

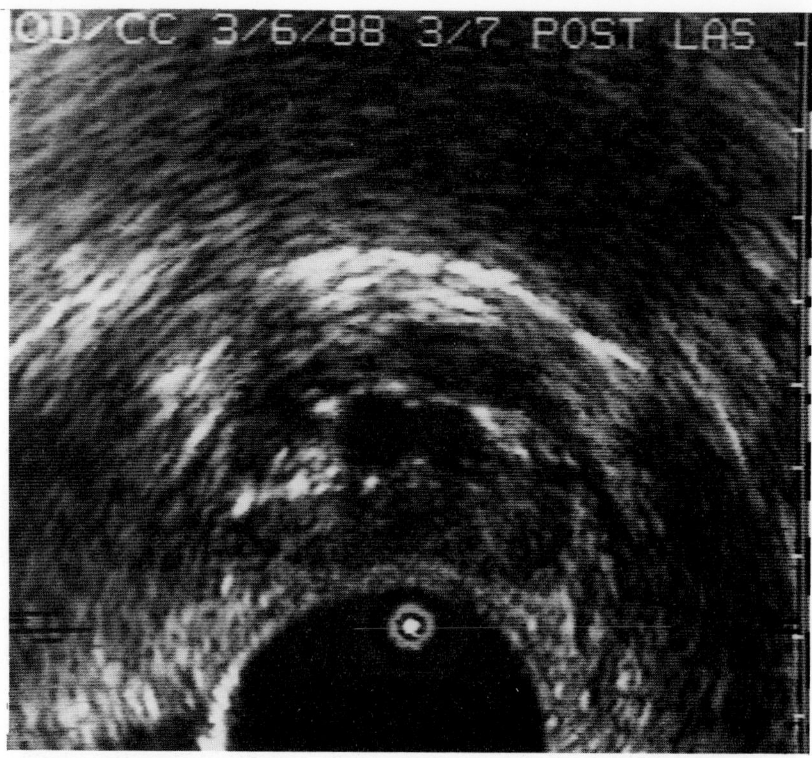

Fig. 4.11. Prostate showing typical laser changes.

Endoscopic liquidization

This is a revolutionary new technique for endoscopically removing prostate tissue using a high-speed mechanical rotating blade. The prostate is liquidized and the resulting solution removed by suction. The endoscopic liquidizer and surgical aspirator (ELSA) can be mechanically guided and the position and amount of tissue removed can be computer-guided by ultrasound images of the gland. The speed of tissue removal is up to 10 g/min. Under ultrasound control, a decent-sized channel in the prostate could be formed in a couple of minutes. This is still at an experimental stage.

Computer-assisted TURP

Both in the United States and China (Chang & Young, 1988), workers have developed a method of teaching resection using computer-assisted imaging of the prostate. The dimensions of the gland are measured by ultrasound, and these measurements are linked to the resectoscope so that the operator never ventures outside certain parameters, i.e. the narrow confines of the prostate. This technique has been successfully applied at the Institute of Urology (Timoney).

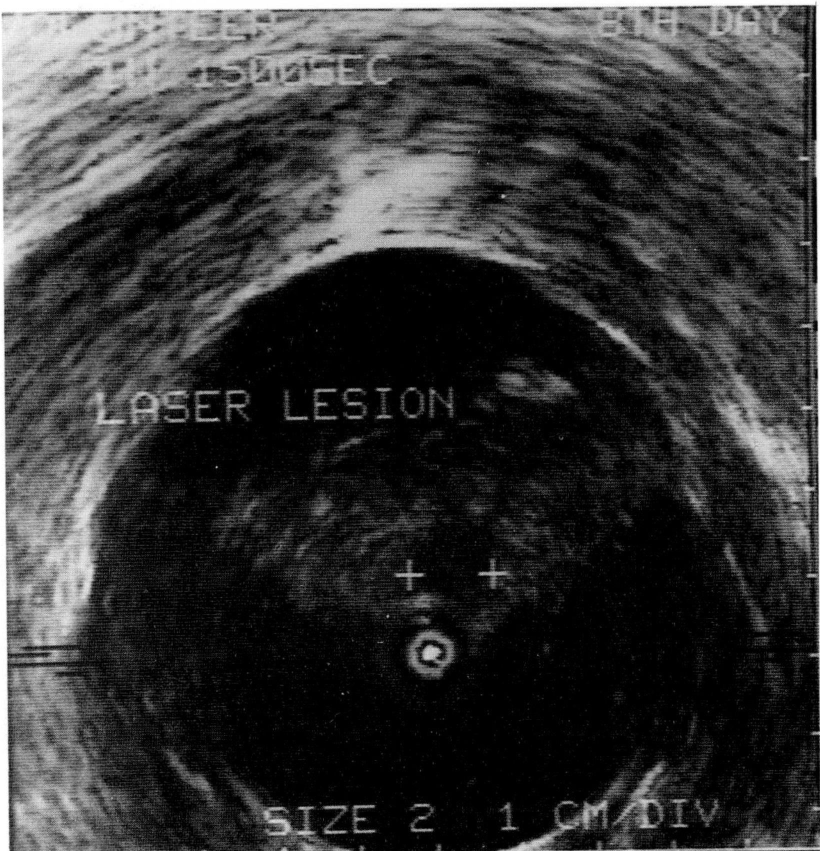

Fig. 4.12. Dog prostate after 1 W for 1500 s.

Conclusion

I hope that in this chapter I have given an insight into the many and varied uses of transrectal ultrasound. Once the users have gained the basic skills of ultrasound, they will find these practical procedures extremely easy to carry out. There is no better modality for imaging the prostate at present, and there is certainly no more accurate method for locating small abnormalities within the prostate gland.

References

Abe M., Hashimoto T., Matsuda T., Saitoh M. & Watanabe H. (1987) Prostatic biopsy guided by transrectal ultrasonography using real-time linear scanner. *Urology,* **29**, 567–9.

Beisland H.O. & Sander S. (1986) First clinical experiences on neodymium-YAG laser irradiation of localized prostate cancer. *Scand. J. Urol. Nephrol.*, **20**, 113–17.

Bergman A., McKenzie C.J., Richmond J., Ballard C.A. & Platt L.D. (1988) Transrectal ultrasound versus cystography in the evaluation of anatomical stress urinary incontinence. *Br. J. Urol.*, **62**, 228–34.

Chang L.S. & Young S.T. (1988) Transurethral prostatectomy with computer-monitored resectoscope. *Br. J. Urol.*, **62**, 54–8.

Green N.A. (1970) Cryosurgery of the prostate gland in the unfit patient. *Br. J. Urol.*, **42**, 10–20.

Holm H.H., Juul N., Pedersen J.F., Hansen H. & Stroyer I. (1983) Transperineal ^{125}iodine seed implantation in prostatic cancer guided by transrectal ultrasonography. *J. Urol.*, **130**, 283–6.

Lee F., Littrup P.J., Kumasaka G.H., Barlaza G.S. & McLeary R.D. (1987) The use of transrectal ultrasound in the diagnosis, guided biopsy, staging and screening of prostate cancer. *Radiographics*, **7**, 627–44.

Lee F., Gray J.M., McLeary R.D., Meadows T.R., Kumasaka G.H. & Borlaza G.S. (1985) Transrectal ultrasound in the diagnosis of prostate cancer: location, echogenicity, histopathology and staging. *The Prostate*, **7**, 117–29.

McNicholas T.A., Carter S.St.C., Wickham J.E.A. & O'Donoghue E.P.N. (1988) YAG laser treatment of early carcinoma of the prostate. *Br. J. Urol.*, **61**, 239–43.

Peeling W.B. & Griffiths G.J. (1984) Imaging of the prostate by ultrasound. *J. Urol.*, **132**, 217–24.

Ragbe H., Aldape H. & Bagley C.M. Jr. (1988) Ultrasound-guided biopsy. Biopty gun superior to aspiration. *Urology*, **32**, 503–6.

Ronstrom L., Tribukait B. & Eposti P.L. (1981) DNA pattern and cytological findings in fine needle apirates of untreated prostatic tumours. A flow-cytometric study. *The Prostate*, **2**, 79–88.

Servadio C., Leib Z. & Lev A. (1987) Diseases of prostate treated by local microwave hyperthermia. *Urology*, **30**, 97–9.

Shabesigh R., Fishman I.J. & Krebs M. (1988) Combined transrectal ultrasonography and urodynamics in the evaluation of detrusor–sphincter dyssynergia. *Br. J. Urol.*, **62**, 326–30.

Von Castenada F., Letourneau J.G., Reddy P., Hulbert J., Hunter D.W. & Castaneda–Zuniga W.R. (1987) Alternative treatment of prostatic urethral obstruction secondary to benign prostatic hypertrophy. *ROFO*, **147**, 426–9.

Watanabe H., Igari D., Tanahashi Y., Harada K. & Saitoh M. *et al.* (1974) Measurements of size and weight of prostate by means of transrectal ultrasonotomography. *Tohoku Journal of Experimental Medicine*, **114**, 277–85.

Watanabe H., Date S., Hiroshi O., Saitoh M. & Tanaka S. (1980) A survey of 3000 examinations by transrectal ultrasonotomography. *The Prostate*, **1**, 271–8.

Whitmore W.F. Jr. (1980) Interstitial radiation therapy for carcinoma of the prostate. *The Prostate*, **1**, 157–68.

5 Balloon dilatation of the prostate

P.F. KEANE

Introduction

The widespread use of balloon dilatation to treat stenoses in arteries and the ureter has led urologists and radiologists to apply balloon dilatation to the prostate and bladder neck to relieve male outflow obstruction. The use of balloons to relieve obstructions in the cardiovascular, gastrointestinal or urological systems offers considerable advantages, namely:

1 the procedure can be performed on an outpatient basis;
2 no general anaesthetic is required;
3 blood transfusion is not required; and
4 significant reduction in cost of treatment.

Dilatation of the prostate as treatment for prostatic hypertrophy is not new. Surgeons in the last century developed instruments to incise the hypertrophied ring of tissue at the bladder neck and thus release the entrapped 'adenoma' (Reddy *et al.*, 1988). In 1910 Hollingworth described manual dilatation of the prostate through a suprapubic approach; however, the first effective transurethral dilatation of the prostate was described by Deisting (1956). He described the results of prostatic dilatation in 324 patients and found that the results were good in more than 90% of patients. Backman (1963) reported that 70% of patients treated with Deisting's dilator were improved at 2 year follow-up but, by 5 years, Sandberg & Sandstrom (1967) reported that 25% of patients required reoperation. At this time transurethral resection of the prostate was becoming the accepted treatment for benign prostatic hypertrophy. It was not until the 1980s with the advent of interventional radiological techniques that interest was once again renewed in dilatation of the prostate.

Burhenne *et al.* (1984) described a study in 10 cadavers in which they dilated the prostatic urethra. As an addendum to this paper Burhenne described how he dilated his own prostate using an 8 mm angioplasty catheter for 30 seconds and found that he had gained significant relief of his nocturia. This was the first report of balloon dilatation of the prostate in a human and the authors envisaged patients performing self-dilatation of the prostate under local anaesthetic on a regular basis.

Experimental studies

Burhenne *et al.* (1984) report a 30–100% widening of the prostatic urethra in human cadavers following dilatation with an 8 mm balloon catheter. Castenada *et al.* (1987) reported the results of balloon dilatation in dogs and found that no significant dilatation of the prostatic urethra occurred when balloons of less than 15 mm were used. The balloons were left inflated for 10 minutes with an internal balloon pressure of between 6 and 8 atmospheres. In 12 dogs in which 20 mm balloons were used there was a significant increase in urethral diameter ranging from 3–4 mm pre-dilatation to 16–18 mm immediately after the dilatation. None of the animals in this study suffered any serious complication. Histological studies on the prostates of these dogs showed ulceration of the urothelium, with subepithelial congestion and focal haemorrhages within the prostate. Prostates removed from dogs 2 weeks after the dilatation showed no specific changes. Quinn *et al.* (1985) reported that the widening of the prostatic urethra of dogs seen after dilatation lasted for up to 6 months.

Patient selection and assessment

Patients with symptoms of outflow obstruction may be considered for balloon dilatation. Clinical examination and careful digital examination of the prostate are essential. Estimation of serum acid phosphatatase and/or prostate specific antigen (PSA) should be done. Free-flow rates should be obtained on two separate occasions and a cystometrogram with pressure flow studies performed if the patient has symptoms of instability. Transrectal ultrasound examination of the prostate with estimation of prostatic volume using serial planimetric measurements is useful if available. Endoscopic assessment of the prostate, bladder neck and bladder is essential. Patients with predominantly 'middle' lobe enlargement are reported to be unsuitable for balloon dilatation because the balloon has the effect of pushing the lobe into the bladder and it can thus return to its original position and act as a ball valve.

Methods

Two sizes of balloon catheter from Meditech™ are in common usage (25 and 30 mm). More recently a 35 mm balloon has become available. Cook™, ASI™ and AMS Optilume also make catheters with various design modifications, such as the use of a bladder balloon to localize the position of the bladder neck before the prostatic balloon is inflated. The present author has experience of the Meditech catheter only. The balloon catheter has a central channel to allow its passage over a guide wire. At either end of the balloon there is a metal ring for radiological identification, which can also be easily visualized with an endoscope (Figs 5.1 and 5.2). At the distal end of the catheter there

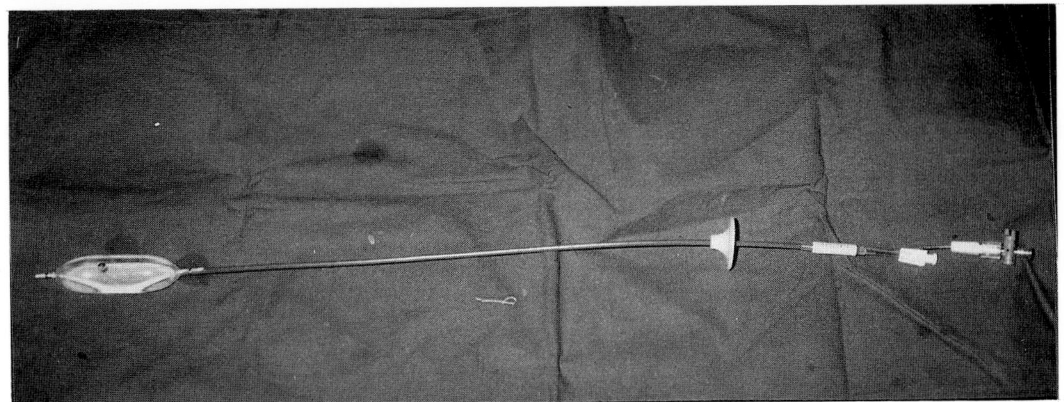

Fig. 5.1. Balloon catheter.

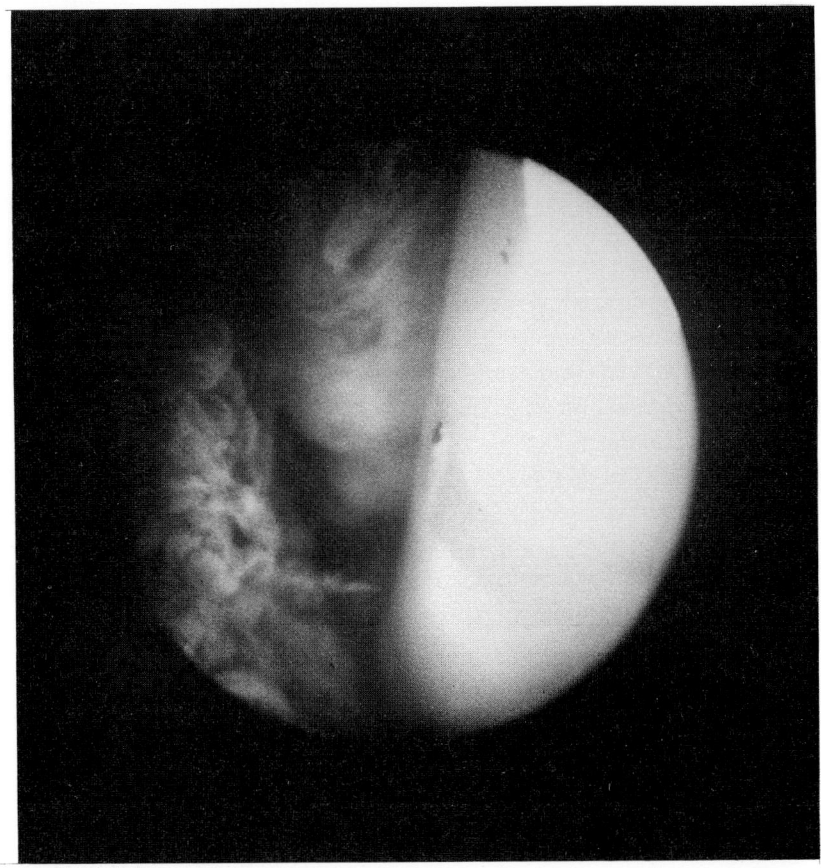

Fig. 5.2. Endoscopic view of the balloon being sited with the verumontanum in the foreground.

is a plastic ring which allows traction to be applied to the balloon during the procedure (Fig. 5.1). Placement of the balloon catheters may be done under sedoanalgesia (pethidine 1 mg/kg and midazolam 0.05–0.1 mg/kg), with 2% lignocaine gel instilled into the urethra 5 minutes before any manipulation or general anaesthesia. In our practice the procedure is covered by a single dose of pre-operative gentamicin.

Endoscopic technique: A floppy-tipped guide wire is passed into the bladder following endoscopic examination of the prostate and bladder. A small-calibre endoscope (rigid or flexible) is then passed beside the catheter and the verumontanum identified. The metal ring of the balloon catheter is placed at the distal end of the verumontanum and the balloon inflated by an assistant while the operator ensures that the balloon is maintained in the correct position. The balloon is inflated with approximately 40 ml of water using a 50 ml syringe. When inflated to maximum, a 10 ml syringe of water is injected into the balloon until firm pressure does not allow the balloon to fill further. This provides approximately 10 atmospheres of pressure within the balloon. The balloon is inflated for 10 minutes and then removed. The patient is catheterized without any need for irrigation, and the catheter remains for 24 hours.

Radiological technique Xylocaine gel (2%) is instilled into the urethra and the patient is given intravenous sedation. A retrograde urethrogram is first performed with the patient in an oblique position and the position of the external sphincter is noted relative to the landmarks of the bony pelvis. It is important that the patient's position be maintained during the procedure. A guide wire is advanced into the bladder and a balloon catheter passed over this, which is then inflated with dilute contrast. The distal marker of the balloon is placed at the distal sphincter as judged by the relative bony landmarks. Check urethrography is performed using a small catheter placed in the urethra alongside the balloon catheter and the use of a penile clamp aids in distension of the bulbar urethra and confirming the position of the sphincter during the procedure. The balloon is inflated for the same period as described above.

All patients will experience a desire to void when the balloon is inflated across the bladder neck, which in some patients may be intense. These patients may require additional sedation; therefore intravenous access is advisable. During the procedure, particularly when performed under radiological screening, there may be some difficulty in maintaining the position of the balloon catheter. As the balloon is inflated the catheter can clearly be felt to be drawn into the bladder and considerable (sometimes alarming) traction has to be applied to keep the balloon in position. The use of a small Foley catheter to screen the position of the catheter is particularly useful and the catheter has to be repositioned a number of times in both the endoscopic and radiological group. We were satisfied in all cases that the catheter was finally positioned correctly.

Results

At the Institute of Urology 13 patients (age range 43–78) with benign prostatic hypertrophy and one patient with a T3 carcinoma of the prostate have now undergone balloon dilatation of the prostate. One patient had had a transurethral resection of his prostate performed 6 years previously. The pre-operative assessment is summarized in Table 5.1. All patients developed bladder spasms with symptoms of urgency and pain after the procedure and two required opiate analgesia within the first 24 hours. All patients had some degree of haematuria but no patient required any intervention. The mean hospital stay was 3.5 days in this series but could be reduced further if the geographical location of the hospital was more convenient for day-case surgery. No patient developed a post-operative urinary tract infection. No patient developed retrograde ejaculation. Patients were seen 3 months after the procedure and free-flow rates were obtained as well as an ultrasound examination of residual urine. The results of the pre-operative urodynamic studies are shown in Table 5.2. Two of the 13 patients in the benign group had a satisfactory result and achieved significant improvement in free-flow rates. One of these patients had a previous transurethral resection of the prostate. The patient with carcinoma of

Table 5.1. Pre-operative assessment

Symptom score
Digital rectal examination
PSA
Flow rate ×2
Residual volume
Cystometry/pressure flow study
Transrectal ultrasound
Endoscopy

Table 5.2. Summary of the pre-operative urodynamic findings

	Prostatic volume	Capacity	End fill pressure	Void pressure	Residual volume
Range	20–66	230–800	12–60	30–120	30–600
Mean	38	458	30	63	108

the prostate experienced significant relief of his symptoms of hesitancy and nocturia (from 5 to 1/night) and his flow rate increased from 3 to 7 ml. There was no significant change in flow characteristics or residual volumes in any of the remaining patients. Nine patients (70%) reported some symptomatic improvement; however, five patients have requested further treatment and three have had transurethral resection of the prostate with satisfactory results.

The results of balloon dilatation in this study from the Institute of Urology (Keane *et al.*, 1990) are the same as those obtained in other centres in the United Kingdom (Gill *et al.*, 1989).

At the Hammersmith Hospital we have recently being using a 35 mm (105 Ch) balloon to treat patients with both outflow obstruction and acute retention of urine. Of 24 patients who presented in retention of urine six were able to void post-operatively. Of the six patients able to void four had flow rates of less than 12 ml/s. All but two patients have been treated by transurethral resection.

Twenty-nine patients with bladder outflow obstruction (BOO) have been treated with the 35 mm balloon and 20 of these had detrusor instability on cystometry. Three month follow-up data is available for 27 of these patients. Twenty-one (78%) had improved flow rates (mean increase 5.3 ml/s) and 19 (70%) had reduced their residual volume (mean reduction 70 ml). Thirteen of the 27 evaluable patients at 3 months were considered unobstructed by pressure flow studies and seven of the 20 patients with detrusor instability had reverted to normal. Overall 19 (70%) of patients noted symptomatic improvement in their symptoms at 3 months. Twelve of 13 patients unobstructed at 3 months returned for urodynamic assessment at 6 months. Only three of the 12 patients were now unobstructed and all experienced deterioration in their urodynamic criteria, however, 10 of the 12 patients continued to be improved symptomatically. The results are summarized in Fig. 5.3.

Many authors have reported that balloon dilatation of the prostate will produce prostatic splitting or commisurotomy and this can be demonstrated on post-operative urethrography (Fig. 5.4). Clinical experience in the United Kingdom (Gill *et al.*, 1989; Keane *et al.*, 1990; McLoughlin *et al.*, 1991) suggests that the presence or absence of commisurotomy has no bearing on the clinical outcome. With the 35 mm balloon 6 of 8 men with commisurotomy were unobstructed when compared with 7 of 12 men without commisurotomy. No patient who was sexually active before the procedure developed retrograde ejaculation and to date there have been no cases of urethral stricture.

Comment

The potential advantages of using balloon dilatation for patients with benign prostatic hypertrophy are that the procedure can be performed without general anaesthesia or blood transfusion and requires minimal

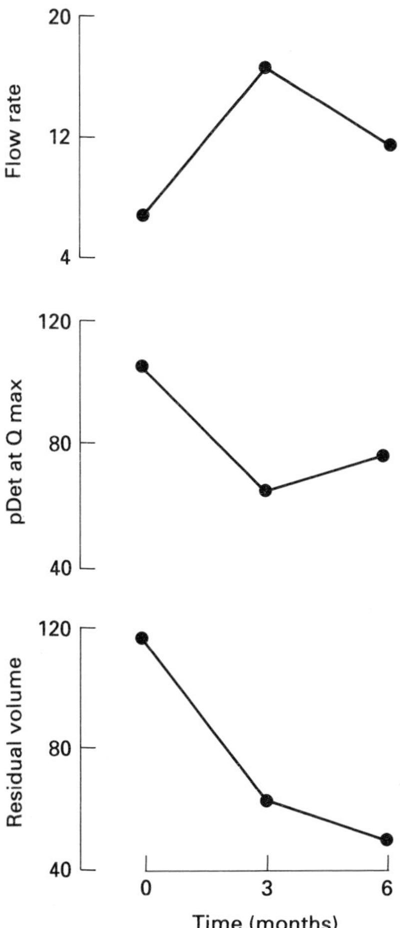

Fig. 5.3. Pre- and post-treatment flow rates, peak detrusor pressure and residual volumes following 35 Ch balloon dilatation.

hospitalization. Also, because the bladder neck is not ablated there is less risk of developing retrograde ejaculation following the procedure.

In animal experiments balloon dilatation of the prostate has been shown to produce intraprostatic haemorrhages but to have no other serious side-effects (Quinn *et al.*, 1985; Castenada *et al.*, 1987). All studies confirm that the procedure is safe and there were no complications in our patients and no sexually active patient developed retrograde ejaculation. Although Castenada *et al.* (1987) and Burhenne *et al.* (1984) report symptomatic improvement in patients there are no objective results reported from these authors. Castenada (1988) reports that 21 of 23 patients with 'lateral lobe' hypertrophy had significant or complete resolution of their symptoms while only five of 12 patients with 'middle lobe' hypertrophy had resolution of symptoms. Fifty per cent of the patients in the Institute of Urology study had symptomatic relief of their symptoms while only 15% had objective

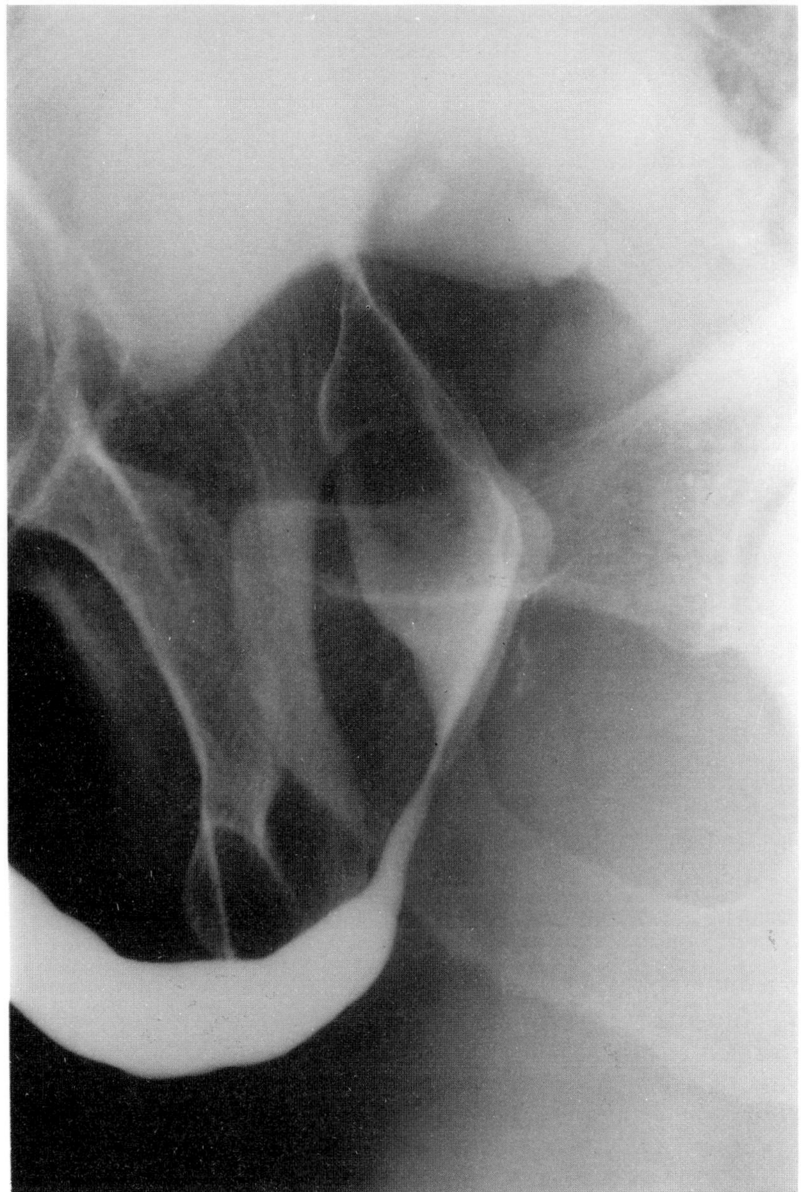

Fig. 5.4. Urethrogram showing a commisurotomy.

improvement in flowmetry. Thus, no firm conclusions can be drawn from the studies presented to date. Table 5.3 summarizes the clinical experience with balloon dilatation in early 1990.

The results of the studies to date indicate that in the majority of patients balloon dilatation of the prostate does not improve objective measurements of outflow obstruction, using either a 25 or a 30 mm balloon. These findings are supported by British workers (pers. comm.). However, symptomatic improvement occurs in 50–70% of patients following balloon dilatation.

Table 5.3. Effects of balloon dilatation on symptoms and objective parameters of outflow obstruction

Author	Year	No.	Balloon size	Symptom improvement	Objective improvement
Perrez*	1989	15	Not stated	80%	8/10
Hulbert*	1989	150	27	60%	Not stated
Klein*	1989	25	Not stated	+	±
Graham*	1989	10	Not stated	50%	No change
Hernandez*	1989	25	25	70%	Not stated
Abrams*	1989	25	25	80%	Not stated
Reddy*	1988	15	25	50%	Not stated
Gill*	1989	48	20/25	54%	11%
Keane*	1990	13	25	50%	No change
McLoughlin*	1990	29	35	70%	Temporary

* *J. Urol.* abstracts AUA meeting Dallas 1989 252A–254A.

Larger balloons (35 mm) are now becoming available and may be more effective than the presently available ones. As discussed above in the series from Hammersmith, 70% of patients had symptomatic improvement and 50% of the patients were unobstructed at 3 months but the results seem to be short-lived and objective parameters of outflow obstruction had reverted to pre-treatment values at 6 months. Larger balloons may be worth evaluation but getting standardized balloon performance at this size is difficult with present technology.

Technique will obviously play an important part in the results obtained but no difference in results obtained using the radiological or the endoscopic techniques were noted in the Institute or Hammersmith series. Malpositioning of the catheter was an unlikely cause for the results presented in these studies. A more plausible explanation is that the benign prostate is quite compliant and can easily accommodate the degree of stretch afforded by this size of balloon catheter and reverts to its normal configuration shortly after the procedure.

Summary

Balloon dilatation of the prostate is not indicated in patients with acute retention. Results with the larger 35 mm balloon are significantly better than those with smaller balloons. With 35 mm balloon dilatation temporary objective improvement can be expected in 50% of patients with symptomatic improvement in up to 70% of patients. Thus the role for balloon dilatation would appear to be mainly in those patients at the extremes of age: for patients presenting with symptoms of bladder outflow obstruction, i.e. younger patients who wish to avoid the effects of surgery on the bladder neck, and those old and infirm patients who wish to avoid the risks of anaesthesia and surgery.

References

Backman K.A. (1963) Dilatation of the prostate according to Deisting. *Acta Chir. Scand,* **126**, 266–74.

Burhenne H.J., Chisholm R.J. & Quenville N.F. (1984) Prostatic hyperplasia: radiological intervention. *Radiology,* **15**, 655–7.

Castenada F., Letourneau J.G., Reddy P., Hulbert J., Hunter D.W., Castenada–Zuniger W.R. & Amplatz K. (1987) Alternative treatment of prostatic urethral obstruction secondary to benign prostatic hypertrophy. *ROFO,* **147**, 426–9.

Castenada F., Lund G., Larson B.W., Limas E., Urness M., Reddy P. & Wasserman N. (1987) Prostatic urethra: experimental dilatation in dogs. *Radiology,* **163**, 645–8.

Castenada W.R. (1988) Non surgical treatment of BPH; prostatic urethroplasty with balloon catheter. Proceedings of the thirteenth annual meeting on Diagnostic Angiography and Interventional Radiology, pp. 230–4, Florida.

Deisting W. (1956) Transurethral dilatation of the prostate. A new method in the treatment of prostatic hypertrophy. *Urol. Int.,* **2**, 158–71.

Gill K.P., Machan L.S., Allison D.J. & Williams G. (1989) Bladder outflow obstruction and urinary retention from prostatic hypertrophy treated by balloon dilatation. *Br. J. Urol.,* **64**, 618–22.

Keane P.F., Charig C., Hudd C., Shah P.J.R., Kellett M.J., Boyle J., Wickham J.E.A. & O'Donoghue E.P.N. (1990) Balloon dilatation of the prostate: Technique and early results. *Br. J. Urol.,* **65**, 354–6.

McLoughlin J., Keane P.F., Jager R., Gill K.P., Machann L. & Williams G. (1991) Dilatation of the prostatic urethra with 35 mm balloon. *Br. J. Urol.,* **67**, 177–18.

Quinn S.F., Dyer R., Smathers R., Glass T., Wright E., Roberts C. & Burke J. (1985) Balloon dilatation of the prostatic urethra. *Radiology,* **157**, 57–61.

Reddy P.K., Wasserman N., Castenada F. & Castenada–Zuniga W.R. (1988) Balloon dilatation of the prostate for treatment of benign hyperplasia. *Urol. Clin. N. Amer.,* **15**, 529–34.

Sandberg I. & Sandstrom B. (1967) Dilatation according to Deisting for prostatic hyperplasia. *Scand. J. Nephrol.,* **1**, 225–6.

6 Prostatic hyperthermia for severe, symptomatic urinary outflow obstruction

A.P. PERLMUTTER AND G.M. WATSON

Introduction

Transurethral resection of hyperplastic prostatic tissue (TURP) is the conventional therapy for urinary outflow obstruction caused by benign prostatic hyperplasia (BPH). This procedure, which results in symptomatic improvement in approximately 75% of patients, requires hospitalization with catheter drainage (Bruskewitz *et al.*, 1986). Complications and side-effects, although seldom severe, include infection, incontinence, retrograde ejaculation, urethral stricture, blood transfusion and impotence. In addition, some patients have severe medical illness which increases anaesthetic and surgical risk.

The disadvantages of TURP have led to the recent development of less invasive interventions. The medical alternatives to resection currently available include anti-androgens and alpha-adrenergic blockade (Caine *et al.*, 1978; Bosch *et al.*, 1989) and 5-alpha-reductase inhibitors are currently under investigation. Medical therapy requires lifelong patient compliance and anti-androgens and alpha-adrenergic blockers can cause significant undesirable side-effects which include erectile dysfunction, orthostatic hypotension and tiredness. This has led to a search for a technique which improves outflow obstruction with a single intervention and minimal morbidity. Transurethral prostatic balloon dilatation requires a general anaesthetic but is a quicker and less traumatic operation than a TURP and preliminary reports are encouraging for some subgroups of patients (Klein & Lemming, 1989). More recently, prostatic hyperthermia has been used without hospitalization to treat patients with urinary outflow obstruction, including those in urinary retention.

The current application of hyperthermia to relieve outflow obstruction has developed from its successful use in treating carcinoma at temperatures from 41 to 45°C. Although the exact mechanism of selective tumour destruction is not known, it is hypothesized that the tumour is less able to dissipate heat than surrounding normal tissue due to a poor blood supply and the inability of malignant vessels to dilate (Song, 1978). Also, the malignant tissue may have an increased sensitivity to heat. The prostate may behave quite differently during heating from malignant tissue and the optimum treatment parameters applicable to BPH and cancer may not be the same. There may be a very large therapeutic difference between treatment at 41 versus 45°C, even though treatment anywhere in this range might be equivalently reported as 'prostatic hyperthermia'.

There are now several hyperthermia devices available and the majority use microwaves to heat the prostate either by a transrectal or transurethral probe. The transurethral applicator is placed into the prostatic urethra as part of a urethral catheter and delivers a circumferential microwave field. The transrectal applicator is placed into the rectum and microwave emission is aimed toward the prostate. In both techniques, the computer-controlled microwave applicator then delivers the amount of energy sufficient to heat the prostate to a target temperature. In some devices the intraprostatic temperatures are directly measured by a urethral catheter containing a thermocouple and other devices calculate the predicted temperature based on the amount of power delivered. Treatment times vary from 50 minutes to 3 hours and the patient may undergo from a single to up to six to ten treatments depending on the device and the protocol being followed. These treatments are performed as outpatients without general or regional anaesthesia. Both the transrectal and transurethral devices are generally well tolerated; however, they are not without patient discomfort. A series of treatments may require multiple urethral catheterizations as well as the placement of an applicator into the rectum. The heating may also be perceived as unpleasant. The patient often experiences a temporary worsening of his obstructive and irritative voiding symptoms in the immediate post-treatment period.

The reported success of these treatments for BPH and acute retention varies widely. There are reports of successful treatments using the transrectal and transurethral devices but there are also reported series demonstrating a lack of efficacy of the technique. Servadio *et al.* (1989) and Lindner *et al.* (1990) report successful patient treatment series with the transurethral and transrectal devices, respectively. However, Strohmaier *et al.* (1990) using the same device as Lindner *et al.* (1990) did not find transrectal treatment efficacious. Part of these discrepancies may lie in the different ways of defining a successful treatment and the difficulty in evaluating subjective symptom data. In addition, treatments at certain temperatures may not be as efficacious as at higher temperatures.

We have treated patients with outflow obstruction due to BPH using three different devices. The Postatherma (Biodan Medical Systems, Rehovot, Israel) heats the prostate by a transrectal applicator with a microwave emission of 915 MHz. There is a cooling system for the rectal wall and a urethral catheter is placed during each treatment to monitor the temperature in the prostatic urethra. The Primus Prostate Machine (Tecnomatix Medical, Antwerp, Belgium) also consists of a transrectal 915 MHz microwave generator and a water cooling system to cool the adjacent rectal mucosa. However, since treatment temperatures are computer-estimated and are not directly measured in the urethra, no catheter is necessary. The Thermex-II (Direx, Technorex Ltd, Petah Tikva, Israel) is a hyperthermia system which heats from inside the prostatic urethra by a heating electrode which is part of a modified Foley catheter. The temperature directly at the heating electrode is sensed by a thermocouple and is considered the maximum treatment temperature.

We have treated patients with outflow obstruction by the above three methods. Follow-up ranges up to 1 year for some of the patients treated with the transrectal devices. Post-treatment peak urinary flow rate, residual urine volume and subjective symptom score are all improved on average. We conclude that the goal of an alternative therapy need not be the attainment of the same flow rate and urodynamic changes found after a TURP but symptomatic improvement so that the patient is once again comfortable with his voiding pattern.

Materials and methods

Patient selection Fifty-five patients who had been refused for treatment with symptoms of BPH for greater than 9 months (mean 1.7 years) were referred for treatment and were included in the study. Nineteen patients were treated with the Prostathermer, 17 with the Primus and 19 with the Thermex-II. All of these patients were candidates for TURP but desired alternative treatment. Initial evaluation included three free urinary flow rates with post-micturition residual urine volumes determined by transabdominal ultrasound, symptom score (Boyarsky *et al.*, 1977) and cystometrogram. All patients had normal upper tracts and did not have urinary lithiasis. Rectal examination, transrectal ultrasound (TRUS) and prostatic specific antigen (PSA) were used to detect prostatic carcinoma and these patients were excluded. The mean patient age in each group was 66 years (Prostathermer), 68 years (Primus) and 66 years (Thermex-II). The mean prostate volumes as determined by TRUS using the Proscan and the ellipsoid approximation volume method were 40 cc (Prostathermer), 38 cc (Primus) and 34 cc (Thermex-II).

The inclusion criteria for the study were: (1) mean peak urinary flow rate < 15 ml/s; (2) cystometrogram findings of outlet obstruction; and (3) patient symptoms which necessitate TURP. Patients with chronic retention were excluded.

Treatment The Biodan Prostathermer treatment protocol consisted of six 1 hour transrectal treatments, at weekly intervals as outpatients. The patients were treated in the semi-lithotomy position and the mean peak temperature attained in our series as measured by the urethral thermocouple was 43°C. A lubricating jelly containing 1%

lignocaine was used for all urethral catheterizations and oral antibiotics were administered at the time of all hyperthermia treatments if a urethral catheter was used.

The Primus treatment protocol also consisted of six 1 hour transrectal treatments, at weekly intervals in the supine position. There was no urethral catheterization. The maximum delivered energy during each treatment was 40 W and the intraprostatic target temperatures calculated by the device were 42.5–44.5°C. This calculated treatment temperature as a function of the power delivered may not be reliable.

The transurethral Thermex-II treatment consisted of a single 3 hour session at 44.5°C. These patients were treated in either the supine or sitting position. The heating electrode is mounted 3 cm from the balloon of a modified Foley catheter and is designed to sit in the prostatic urethra when the balloon is at the bladder neck. Since the localization of the heating unit in the prostate necessitates that the balloon is at the bladder neck, the catheter is secured on gentle traction after 10 ml of water is instilled in the balloon. The intraprostatic placement of the metal thermocouple was verified using transrectal ultrasound.

In general, all patients were assessed at 6, 26 and 52 weeks by flow rate and post-micturition residual urine volume, transrectal prostatic ultrasound and symptom score. None of the patients who started the study have been lost to follow-up. The objective and subjective data for those patients who have gone on to have a prostatectomy are included only for those follow-up visits prior to having surgery.

Results

All patients tolerated the treatments reasonably well and completed the series of six Prostathermer or Primus transrectal sessions. Two Thermex-II treatments needed to be prematurely terminated.

There was no change in prostatic volume or appearance as measured by TRUS after either of the two types of transrectal treatments. The mean pre- and post-treatment volumes for the patients treated with the Prostathermer were 45 cc and 41 cc respectively and 38 cc and 37 cc respectively for those treated with the Primus. Similarly, there was no change in the volumes of those treated with the transurethral Thermex-II: 34 cc pre-treatment and 30 cc after treatment. However, at 6 weeks post-treatment, four of the 19 Thermex-II patients developed new small, scattered, periurethral intraprostatic hyperechoic regions. This had not been observed on any of the patients treated with the transrectal devices. The initial prostatic volume did not correlate with the degree of subjective or objective patient response.

Table 6.1 summarizes the change in mean peak urinary flow rate for the three treated groups. The post-therapy flow rate is determined 6 weeks after the last treatment. We found that all three groups on average experienced an increase in their peak mean urinary free-flow rate. The increase from 7.3 ml/s to 10.6 ml/s at 6 week post-

Table 6.1. Changes in mean peak urinary flow rate

Treatment modality	Pre-therapy (ml/s)	6 weeks post-therapy (ml/s)	6–12 months post-therapy (ml/s)
Prostathermer	7.3 ± 2.1	10.6 ± 3.4	11.0 ±3.1
Primus	7.8 ± 3.5	10.4 ± 3.4	10.3 ± 3.2
Thermex-II	8.9 ± 3.0	9.6 ± 3.0	—

Flow rates are expressed ± SD. There is no 6–12 month follow-up on the Thermex-II group.

Prostathermer treatment was sustained at the 1 year follow-up visit at 11.0 ml/s. Similarly, the Primus group had an increase in mean peak flow rate from 7.8 ml/s to 10.4 ml/s at 6 weeks post-treatment and this remained constant at 10.3 ml/s at the 6 month follow-up. The Thermex-II group had the smallest increase in flow rate from 8.9 ml/s to 9.6 ml/s at 6 weeks. The Thermex-II patients do not yet have 6 month follow-up.

Table 6.2 shows the reduction in post-micturition residual urine volume for the three treated groups. The Prostathermer group started with the largest mean residual volume of 159 ml and this went to 71 ml at 6 weeks and 60 ml at 1 year. The Primus group similarly decreased from 112 ml pre-treatment to 30 ml post-treatment and 38 ml at 6 months post-treatment. The Thermex-II group started with the lowest residual urine volume but, even from this starting 82 ml residual, a decrease to 62 ml was found at 6 weeks post-treatment.

Table 6.3 summarizes the change in subjective symptom score for the three groups (Boyarsky *et al.*, 1977). This scoring system includes nocturia, daytime frequency, hesitancy, intermittency, terminal dribbling, urgency, impairment of size and force of stream, dysuria, and the sensation of incomplete bladder emptying. Each symptom is scored from 0 to 3 depending on precisely defined criteria for the severity of

Table 6.2. Changes in post-micturition residual urine volume

Treatment modality	Pre-therapy (ml)	6 weeks post-therapy (ml)	6–12 months post-therapy (ml)
Prostathermer	159 ± 105	71 ± 47	60 ± 57
Primus	112 ± 92	30 ± 63	38 ± 60
Thermex-II	82 ± 61	62 ± 27	—

Urine volume is expressed ± SD. There is no 6–12 month follow-up on the Thermex-II group.

Table 6.3. Changes in patient symptom score

Treatment modality	Pre-therapy	6 weeks post-therapy	6–12 months post-therapy
Prostathermer	12 ± 2.2	6 ± 3.1	7 ± 2.8
Primus	11 ± 2.9	7 ± 3.2	9 ± 3.1
Thermex–II	11 ± 3.4	9 ± 2.9	—

Symptom scores are expressed ± SD, and are calculated by the method of Boyarsky *et al.* (1977). There is no 6–12 month follow-up on the Thermex-II group.

each symptom. The three prostatic heating techniques each had a large impact on patient symptomatic score and this remains improved at the 6 month and 1 year follow-up. The patients on average have a much improved voiding pattern and this is evident in their subjective symptoms.

In general, the treatments were well tolerated but do involve discomfort. Most patients treated with the transrectal devices experienced the urge to void due to mild bladder spasm but neither medication nor the cessation of treatments was necessary. More severe bladder spasms occurred in approximately one-third of Thermex-II patients necessitating machine restarts and one treatment to be prematurely terminated. The rectal applicator itself and the perineal warmth due to the heating become uncomfortable by the end of the 1 hour Primus and Prostathermer sessions. The multiple urethral catheterizations needed for the Prostathermer can be similarly difficult for the patient. The majority of patients treated with the Prostathermer had mild transient haematuria but this was only experienced by a few of the Primus and Thermex-II group. Dysuria was associated with almost all catheterized patients and resolved within 2–3 days after treatments.

Complications and treatment failures are shown in Table 6.4. Four Prostathermer (21%) and two Thermex-II (12%) patients developed urinary tract infection despite 24 hours of peri-procedure oral antibiotic coverage. Acute urinary retention occurred in three Prostathermer patients (16%), two of whom were concomitantly infected, and three Thermex-II (16%) patients without urinary infection. All of these episodes resolved after catheter decompression for 1 to 7 days and the treatment of infection when present. Most patients treated with the transrectal devices experienced some post-treatment rectal burning but two patients treated both with the Prostathermer (11%) and the Primus (12%) complained of rectal burning which persisted for many days. One Prostathermer (5%) and two Thermex-II (11%) patients experienced syncope during treatment, most likely brought on by treatment discomfort and bladder spasm. The Primus group, which did not undergo urethral catheterization, did not experience

Table 6.4. Complications and treatment failures

Complication	Prostathermer ($n = 19$)	Primus ($n = 17$)	Thermex-II ($n = 19$)
UTI alone	2 (11%)	0	2 (11%)
Retention and UTI	2 (11%)	0	0
Retention without UTI	1 (5%)	0	3 (16%)
Rectal discomfort	0	2 (12%)	0
Syncope	1 (5%)	0	2 (11%)
TURP	2 (11%)	2 (12%)	0

any urinary infection or retention and in general had the fewest complications.

None of the patients have been lost to follow-up and further evaluation is ongoing. Only four patients have had a prostatectomy. The remainder of the patients (93%) are currently no longer candidates for TURP or are still deciding if they are content with current symptoms.

Discussion

The term hyperthermia has become associated with the current trend for heat treatment of the prostate but it has is origin in the treatment of malignant tissue. Indeed the initial experience with the transrectal microwave probe was in prostatic cancer. Hyperthermia aims to treat malignant tissue at temperatures of 41–44.5°C at which temperature the malignant tissue is supposedly more susceptible than benign tissue (Song, 1978). Therapy therefore demanded a very careful monitoring of the temperature profile across the region. When this modality came to be assessed in BPH therapy, the approach was at best empirical. There is no reason to suppose that a benign prostatic adenoma will respond in the same way as malignant tissue. This discussion will consider the published literature and compare the different treatment conditions and methods. Our results will be compared with other series and the placebo effect will be considered. Finally, a therapeutic context for hyperthermia will be proposed.

The Biodan Prostathermer transrectal microwave experience

The first use of microwave hyperthermia for the treatment of BPH was published by Yerushalmi *et al.* (1985). They treated a group of 11 patients in urinary retention and 18 with severe outflow obstruction who were considered unfit for prostatectomy with a transrectal hyperthermia device. Temperatures of 42–43°C were measured in the prostatic urethra within 10–15 minutes of starting treatment. They found that all treated patients with obstructive symptoms showed some degree of subjective improvement and eight of 11 patients in retention were able to void satisfactorily after treatment.

This preliminary success encouraged Servadio *et al.* (1986) to develop further the use of a transrectal probe, the Biodan Prostathermer, for BPH clinically. In their main study of 140 patients with outflow obstruction the mean peak urinary flow rate of the whole group improved from 10.1 ml/s pre-treatment to 14.1 ml/s and 11.9 ml/s at 3 and 6 months respectively (Servadio *et al.*, 1989). Treatment temperatures were 42 ± 1°C. The post-micturition residual urine volume fell from 180 ml to 101 ml and 90 ml at 3 and 6 months respectively. The group, however, included many different treatment protocols and some patients received cyproterone acetate (although this may have been during the treatment only). Lindner *et al.* (1990) have used the Prostathermer to treat 72 patients at 42 ± 1.5°C who had failed a trial of catheter removal after going into acute retention. By 1 month, 50% were freed of their catheters and at 1 year 40% were still free. Again cyproterone acetate was used but only during the course of treatment. Saranga *et al.* (1990) treated 83 severely obstructed patients at 42.5 ± 1°C with the Prostathermer and noted that 42% had objective improvement. The mean flow rate of the group as a whole improved from 10.2 ml/s pre-treatment to 12.7 ml/s and 12.1 ml/s at 3 and 6 months respectively. The residual fell from 130 ml to 42 ml and 46 ml at 3 and 6 months. In addition there were 31 patients in acute retention of which 61% were able to dispense with their catheters post-treatment. The authors' argument that these improvements at least in the patients not in acute retention may fall within the range of the improvements which occur in patients included in the placebo arms of controlled trials will be reviewed later. The mean peak flow rate and residual urine volume improvements reported by the above groups are quite similar to our Prostathermer series.

Strohmaier *et al.* (1990) expressed profound disappointment using the Prostathermer at 42–43°C because it did not combine the advantages of reduced prostatic bulk and increased flow which is seen in successful transurethral resection. He did not find any significant improvement in flow rate or residual urine volume in 21 of 23 treated patients. However, 54% of these patients reported subjective improvement in voiding symptoms, 46% did not. They discount the importance of subjective improvement and report a success rate of 7.1%. Only one of five patients in retention could void after treatment. They are at a loss to explain the discrepancy to the above-reported studies except they note that their patient population was younger (65 versus 76 years). Zerbib *et al.* (1990) have reported the only controlled study to date comparing the treatment with a sham group where the temperature rise was insignificant. Their results in their final presentation (although only alluded to in their abstract) suggested a significantly greater improvement in the treated group compared with the sham group.

The Primus versus the Biodan

The Primus system uses an identical wavelength to the Biodan system but does not use a urethral catheter. In the Biodan system the catheter incorporates a receiving antenna which facilitates alignment of a rectal applicator and which also incorporates a series of urethral thermocouples which give some indication of the intraprostatic temperatures. Newman and Knapp (1990) showed that the calculated maximum intraprostatic temperature bore a close relationship to the recorded maximum temperature but that this bore no relationship to the delivered power from the rectal applicator. The Primus system does not employ a urethral catheter and the calculated intraprostatic temperatures are calculated from the power delivered. These temperatures therefore may not be realistic. In practice, however, this apparent defect does not seem to detract from the clinical efficacy. Accurate temperature measurements are a *sine qua non* of a properly conducted hyperthermia treatment but as intimated earlier there is no sound basis for supposing that BPH tissue behaves in the same manner as frank malignant tissue.

Van Erps *et al.* (1990) treated 23 patients who had outflow obstruction with the Primus and found that 56% showed subjective improvement and the mean peak flow rate increased from 7.9 ml/s to 14.3 ml/s. Our Primus results are similar for subjective parameters but show less flow-rate increase. We found no change in prostatic volumes on transrectal ultrasound pre- and post-treatment. Strohmaier *et al.* (1990) and Saranga *et al.* (1990) confirm that the prostatic size remains unaltered. When results of most series are compared, there is little difference between the Primus and the Biodan (40 W compared with 42–44°C). However, the Primus does have the advantage of fewer complications.

Thus the transrectal effect (if any) is not due to shrinkage of the prostate secondary to hyperthermia but rather is due to some subtle change — possibly in the muscular component of the obstruction corresponding to alpha-blockade. Presumably there is a threshold temperature at which this effect occurs but there may well be wide tolerance in the maximum therapeutic temperature. Both the Biodan and the Primus systems deliver up to 40 W. Therefore they share the same limitations in whether or not they can achieve the threshold for the therapy. The only significant difference between the systems is that with the Primus some areas of the prostate may exceed 44.5°C. The fact that this is probably not a disadvantage is borne out by the lack of complications using the Primus system.

The transurethral versus the transrectal approach

The transrectal approach is relatively inefficient because a significant proportion of the microwave power is lost in heating the water used to cool the rectal wall. The microwaves have to penetrate tissues with different densities and reflections may well occur at interfaces, especially that between the perirectal fat and the prostate. Newman & Knapp (1990) found that with the transrectal approach the part of the prostate anterior to the urethra was heated above body temperature but well below maximum treatment temperature. A probe inserted transurethrally can be positioned accurately and easily. One can then have some confidence that the centre of the prostate will achieve the temperature intended. The Thermex-II system has been used in this study in a small number of patients.

We found that in our Thermex-II patients improvements in peak urinary flow rate and post-micturition residual urine volumes have occurred, but have been slight. In the transrectal-treated patients who have so far come to TURP, there have been no changes detectable on light microscopy of the prostatic chips. In contrast, we have found there has been evidence of infarction in the periurethral tissue after Thermex-II treatment. Transurethral techniques may therefore act both by reducing the static obstructive element of the glandular tissue and by some possible effect on the muscular component of the obstruction. The treatment schedule with the Thermex-II is also attractive because patients can be treated two at a time in single or possibly two sessions lasting 3 hours each. Other than treatment schedule convenience, our early results with this technique have failed to show any superiority of the transurethral device over the transrectal systems in practice.

Sapozink *et al.* (1990) have reported on the use of their BSD probe (BSD Medical, Salt Lake City, Utah). This is a microwave probe, with 630 or 925 MHz delivered transurethrally. The treatment schedule is up to 10 treatments of 1 hour with temperatures reaching as high as 47.5°C. They reported on 21 patients with a flow rate increase from 11.0 ml/s to 15.9 ml/s and a residual urine volume decrease from 177 ml to 91 ml. The average size of the prostates in this group was 97 cc which fell to 79 cc after therapy. This shrinkage in prostatic volume is corroborated by the demonstration of histological changes in the periurethral region (Baert *et al.*, 1990). The group treated in Sapozink *et al.*'s series had a significantly different prostatic size from that in our series where the average prostatic volume was 34 cc. The prostatic sizes in Sapozink's patients ranged from 34 cc to 301 cc and therefore TURP would not have been practicable in some of these patients.

The Prostatron (Technomed International) is also a transurethral microwave device. It stands out in two ways: it is considerably more expensive than the other devices and it combines a cooling system to preserve the prostatic urethra while heating the deeper prostatic tissue.

Carter *et al.* (1990) have reported on 24 patients with outflow obstruction and 12 patients with acute retention who have been treated by a single 50 minute session on the Prostatron with 30–45 W of peak power delivered. Peak urinary flow rate increases of greater than 4 ml/s were seen in 62% of patients at 3 months post-treatment. Two of nine patients in the earlier part of their experience and two of three patients in the later part of their experience (when higher temperatures were achieved) have been freed of their catheters. Devonec *et al.* (1990) treated patients with this device prior to radical surgery in order to assess the zone of heat damage. They reported evidence of heat damage up to 17 mm from the urethra but with preservation of the urethra within a distance of 2–5 mm.

Thus transurethral devices do have the potential of causing necrosis and therefore acting on the static as well as the dynamic component of obstruction. This is in contrast to the lack of any histological change found upon examination of prostatic tissue after treatment with the transrectal devices. It is a slightly more invasive procedure than the simple application of just a rectal applicator as with the Primus system. Certainly the results with the BSD device are impressive, especially when the prostatic sizes are taken into consideration. However, the BSD device does have the drawback of requiring six to 10 treatment sessions. The Prostatron's short, single session is appealing, and the Thermex-II device has the advantage of being extremely practical in that two patients can be treated at one time. However, the adoption of single-session protocols may have more to do with marketing strategy than with clinical experience.

It is not entirely clear why the Prostatron system has incorporated urethral cooling so that the prostatic urothelium is spared. Certainly there does not seem to be any problem with sloughing or bleeding associated with the BSD or Thermex-II treatments. Mebust & White (1977) used a metal plate attached to a high-frequency current to 'desiccate' the prostate. They reported that a few patients developed symptoms compatible with chronic prostatitis. Perhaps it was felt in some way that preserving the urethra would protect against this complication. However, there have not yet been reports of prostatitis-like symptoms with either the transrectal or transurethral devices.

The importance of treatment temperature and time

The optimum treatment temperatures for BPH are not known and the range of temperatures previously used for hyperthermia of carcinoma have been empirically adopted. Leib *et al.* (1986) examined canine prostate tissue after microwave treatment at temperatures ranging from 40 to 47°C. They found that permanent histological change was time- and temperature-dependent. Treatment at 42.5 ± 0.5°C up to 1.5 hours results in a mononuclear inflammatory infiltration but this is transient and treatment at this temperature could be repeated multiple times without permanent change. Although harmless, is this the ideal therapeutic temperature? In contrast, treatment at 44.5 ± 0.5°C for 1.5 hours results in necrosis of the prostatic urethra, haemorrhage and inflammatory infiltration. This canine study is similar to our observations that the transrectal approach, which is generally heating to 42.5°C, shows no histopathological change, whereas transurethral heating to 44.5°C causes histological change. Sapozink *et al.* (1990) in many ways report the most successful series and they had occasional peak treatment temperatures of 47.5°C.

Since both approaches yield similar preliminary clinical results in our hands, what can be concluded about treatment temperature? It may be that the necrosis at the higher temperature is not part of the therapeutic effect. However, since the necrosis brings about permanent histological change, it is possible that longer follow-up will reveal a difference between the methods. Forty-two degrees might be on the verge of effective temperature and may explain the difference in effectiveness reported above for the Prostathermer in different series. Finally, the treatment time regimens and the maximum treatment temperatures currently in use are effective, but neither of these parameters has yet been optimized.

Final discussion

There are a number of issues which are raised when considering any new modality for the treatment of BPH. The first of these is the proper assessment of whether the technique is really efficacious. The placebo response is well known and in addition some patients spontaneously improve. Ball *et al.* (1981) followed 107 patients with outflow obstruction proven on cystometography but without symptoms severe enough to warrant a TURP. Thirty per cent reported a subjective improvement on no treatment at all and only 10% deteriorated sufficiently to require surgery. Resnick *et al.* (1983) demonstrated a statistically significant improvement in subjective symptoms as well as peak urinary flow rates in a placebo group participating in a controlled drug study. Issacs (1990) has reviewed a number of patients, including those of Ball *et al.*, and found that approximately 20% tend to improve and 20% tend to deteriorate after initial evaluation. The spontaneous improvements all tended to occur in patients with a history of symptoms of 6 months or less and was rare in any patient who had had symptoms for more than 6 months. All of the patients in our series gave histories with symptoms lasting 9 months or more. Further, according to Isaacs (1990) the placebo effect as seen in the placebo arms of drug trials is never prolonged and symptoms tend to revert to baseline by 6 months. This argument suggests that there is a placebo effect in the patients treated with some of the microwave devices, but follow-up of 6 months or greater will diminish its importance. Carefully constructed clinical trials comparing sham to real treatments need to be performed to confirm this.

A second issue is that those patients who avoid TURP will also not have a careful histological examination of the prostatic chips. Current evaluation of the prostate by rectal palpation, transrectal ultrasound and PSA is still limited and some patients with occult carcinoma will therefore not be identified. It may, therefore, prove necessary to continue following up patients after these alternative therapies just in case of occult carcinoma. Those treatments which produce frank necrosis within the prostate may cause abnormal areas on transrectal ultrasound scans which may in turn lead to unnecessary biopsies. Perhaps the issue should be resolved by performing four quadrant biopsies of the prostate prior to treatment.

Our experience with prostatic hyperthermia has been on patients with sufficiently severe outflow obstruction to justify prostatectomy in each case. After therapy the majority of our patients have been improved sufficiently so that they no longer require treatment. The patients were actively seeking this treatment and were highly motivated to avoid surgery in most instances. Therefore, it is important that this study be repeated on patients who present to standard urological clinics. It may be that the symptomatic improvement that such a patient experiences will prove inadequate if that patient is not strongly trying to avoid surgery. We can only conclude from our study that only two out of 19 patients came to TURP after treatment with the Biodan device and two out of 17 patients treated with the Primus device. Our experience with the Thermex-II device is too short for comment at this moment. The majority of the patients who have not come to surgery are sufficiently improved both objectively and subjectively that they no longer wish to be considered for the operation. However, we base this more on their absence of symptoms than on the fact that they are no longer obstructed. Follow-up cystometrography is being performed on our patients and our impression at this moment is that they remain obstructed. There are at most small improvements on cystometrography. Therefore, routine patient follow-up including upper tract evaluation remains essential.

Transrectal hyperthermia appears to improve patients objectively and subjectively without causing necrosis of the gland. It is, therefore, possibly acting in a manner similar to alpha-blockers. If this is the case then the next question is whether transrectal devices actually are superior to alpha-blockers. A trial comparing transrectal hyperthermia with alpha-blockers should be conducted. Transurethral techniques have the potential for causing necrosis, although in our early experience with the Thermex-II device we have not demonstrated any superiority of this device over transrectal hyperthermia. There is probably greater potential for the development of transurethral devices for creating the sort of cavity which can be achieved by a TURP. The advantage of such a transurethral device would be in cost and in that the treatment would be completely done as an outpatient and without blood loss. TURP would be reserved as a first-line treatment for patients with chronic retention or particularly large middle lobes. Prostatic hyperthermia is not a replacement for TURP, and should not be considered as such. However, even though the patient remains obstructed, the objective and most importantly subjective improvement allows certain patients to attain a satisfactory voiding pattern which obviates the need for more invasive surgical intervention.

Although these treatments are much less invasive than a TURP, they are not without complication and patient discomfort. Treatment with the transrectal applicator becomes uncomfortable at the end of an hour session and many patients find the feeling of perineal warmth quite bothersome. Each Prostathermer involves a urethral catheterization as well. The initial part of the Thermex-II treatment is characterized by a rapid temperature rise to 44.5°C and the first part of this session is often painful due to the heat or associated bladder spasm. Most, but not all, of these patients adapt to the prostatic heating and it no longer is perceived as painful only 10 minutes into the treatment.

We are, therefore, looking towards ways of increasing the efficacy of existing devices and also looking at laser techniques in order to try to minimize surgical intervention. Our other aim is to develop an algorithm so that any particular features, such as a large middle lobe on vesical ultrasound, could be used to identify which is the most appropriate treatment modality. In the meantime we can at least say that the existing techniques appear to be useful and patient satisfaction is high but with relatively little improvement to the obstruction for the investment of time which needs to be made. The fact that we are at an early stage in the evolution of applying high technology to the prostate should not be an excuse for ignoring these developments. The technology exists for providing a sizeable central cavity in the prostate gland.

References

Baert L., Ameye F., Astrahan M. & Petrovich Z. (1993) Transurethral microwave hyperthermia for benign prostatic hyperplasia, the Leuven experience. *J. Endourol.*, **7**, 61–9.

Ball A.J., Feneley R.C.L. & Abrams P.H. (1981) The natural history of untreated 'prostatism'. *Br. J. Urol.*, **53**, 613–16.

Bosch R.J.L.H., Griffiths D.J., Blom J.H.M. & Schroeder F.H. (1989) Treatment of benign prostatic hyperplasia by androgen deprivation: effects on prostate size and urodynamic parameters. *J. Urol.*, **141**, 68–72.

Boyarsky S., Jones G., Paulson D.F. & Prout G.R. (1977) A new look at bladder neck obstruction by the Food and Drug Administration regulators: Guidelines for investigation of benign prostatic hypertrophy. *Trans. Am. Assoc. Genito-Urin. Surg.*, **68**, 29–32.

Bruskewitz R.C., Larsen E.H., Madsen P.O. & Dorflinger T. (1986) Three year follow-up of urinary symptoms after transurethral resection of the prostate. *J. Urol.*, **136**, 613–5.

Caine M., Perlberg S. & Meretyk S. (1978) A placebo-controlled double-blind study of the effect of phenoxybenzamine in benign prostatic obstruction. *Br. J. Urol.*, **50**, 551–4.

Carter S., Patel A., Ramsey J., Perrin P. & Devonec M. (1990) Objective clinical results of transurethral microwave thermometry for benign prostatic obstruction. *J. Endourol.*, **4**, 134 (Suppl.).

Devonec M., Cathaud M., Carter S., Berger N. & Perrin P. (1990) Transurethral microwave therapy in patients with benign prostatic hypertrophy. *J. Endourol.*, **4**, 135 (Suppl.).

Issacs J.T. (1990) Importance of the natural history of benign prostatic hyperplasia in the evaluation of pharmacologic intervention. *Prostate Suppl.*, **3**, 1–7.

Klein L.A. & Lemming B. (1989) Balloon dilatation for prostatic obstruction. Long term follow-up. *Urology*, **33**, 198–201.

Leib Z., Rothem A., Lev A. & Servadio C. (1986) Histopatholocal observations in the canine prostate treated by local microwave hyperthermia. *The Prostate*, **8**, 93–102.

Lindner A., Braf Z., Lev A. *et al.* (1990) Local hyperthermia of the prostate gland for the treatment of benign prostatic hypertrophy and urinary retention. *Br. J. Urol.*, **65**, 201–3.

Mebust W.K. & White T.G. (1977) Immune reactions following desiccation surgery of the canine prostate: an initial report. *Invest. Urol.*, **14**, 427–30.

Newman D. & Knapp P. (1990) Interstitial temperature mapping in human prostate during transrectal hyperthermia treatment for BPH. *J. Endourol.*, **4**, 135 (Suppl.).

Resnick M.I., Jackson J.E., Watts L.E. & Boyce W.H. (1983) Assessment of the antihypercholesterolemic drug, probucol, in benign prostatic hyperplasia. *J. Urol.*, **129**, 206–9.

Sapozink M.D., Boyd S.D., Astrahan M.A., Jozsef G. & Petrovich Z. (1990) Transurethral hyperthermia for benign prostatic hyperplasia: preliminary clinical results. *J. Urol.*, **113**, 944–50.

Saranga R., Matzkin H. & Braf Z. (1990) Local microwave hyperthermia in the treatment of benign prostatic hyperplasia. *Br. J. Urol.*, **65**, 349–53.

Servadio C., Leib Z. & Lev A. (1986) Further observations on the use of local hyperthermia for the treatment of diseases of the prostate in man. *Eur. J. Urol.*, **12**, 38–40.

Servadio C., Linder A., Lev A., Leib Z., Siegel Y. & Braf Z. (1989) Further observations on the effect of local hyperthermia on benign enlargement of the prostate. *World J. Urol.*, **6**, 204–8.

Song C.W. (1978) Effect of hyperthermia on vascular functions of normal tissues and experimental tumours. *J. Nat. Cancer Inst.*, **60**, 711–13.

Strohmaier W.L., Bichler K.H., Fluchter S.H. & Wilbert D.M. (1990) Local microwave hyperthermia of benign prostatic hyperplasia. *J. Urol.*, **144**, 913–17.

Van Erps P., Dourcy B. & Denis L.J. (1990) Transrectal hyperthermia in benign prostatic hyperplasia (BPH). *Abstracts Eur. Assoc. Urol.*, **IX**, Congress 18 (Suppl. 1), 510.

Yerushalmi A., Fishelovitz Y., Singer D. *et al.* (1985) Localized deep microwave hyperthermia in the treatment of poor operative risk patients with benign prostatic hyperplasia. *J. Urol.*, **133**, 873–6.

Zerbib M., Steg A. & Conguy S. (1990) A prospective randomized study of localized hyperthermia vs. placebo in obstructive benign hypertrophy of the prostate. *J. Urol.*, **143** (Suppl.), 284A.

7 Chronic prostatitis: a functional voiding disturbance?

D.G. BARNES

Introduction

Young & Davies in their 1926 classic treatise on urology extensively described the condition of chronic prostatitis. This condition was commonly thought to be a complication of gonorrhoea and generally thought to be infective in nature. The patient complained of an urethral discharge, dysuria with frequency or urgency, and local prostatic, perineal or rectal pain, which was also referred to other regions of the body. Pain on ejaculation and other sexual symptoms such as impotence also occurred. The diagnosis was confirmed by clinical examination and the recovery of excess pus cells and bacteria from the prostatic fluid, produced by prostatic massage. Treatment consisted of frequent prostatic massage, the instillation of intraurethral antiseptics and reassurance. The outcome of treatment was then, as now, generally poor. This was attributed to 'rebellious infections' which resisted ordinary treatments.

Patients complaining of painful symptoms attributed to the prostate gland are still a frequent chronic problem in the urological outpatients' department. In order to aid treatment and investigation leading workers in this field suggested a classification based on the Stamey bacterial localization technique (Meares & Stamey, 1968; Drach *et al.*, 1978). They categorized patients according to microscopic and bacteriological findings into chronic bacterial prostatitis, abacterial prostatitis and prostatodynia, whereas on clinical grounds alone it is often impossible to separate these groups of patients.

Response to specific treatment on the whole is still poor and the condition often runs a relapsing course. This explains the plethora of remedies which have been utilized. These include antibiotics, both systemic and local, anti-inflammatory preparations including steroids, alpha-adrenergic blockade, striated muscle relaxants, prostatic decongestants, pollen extracts, repeated prostatic massage, prostatectomy including radical surgery, heat in the form of the sitz bath, and most recently transrectal microwave-induced hyperthermia. In the chronic case, the outcome of treatment is often poor, unless the diagnosis is based on recurrent urinary tract infections, the source of which having been localized to the prostate gland. This rare group of patients has been extensively studied (Meares & Stamey, 1972; Meares,

A functional voiding disturbance?

1977), including immunological response to the infecting organism (Shortliffe *et al.*, 1980, 1981), which is usually a Gram-negative bacillus, e.g. *Escherichia coli*. These patients respond to appropriate antibiotics and are relatively asymptomatic between attacks. In the commoner group, symptoms of perineal, penile, testicular, rectal and suprapubic pain associated with an alteration in the voiding pattern wax and wane regardless of treatment. This poor response has been attributed to poor bacteriological screening, poor penetration of antibiotics into the prostatic fluid and delayed commencement of appropriate treatment (Stamey *et al.*, 1970). An alternative explanation is that this group of conditions are not entirely infective in origin and other aetiological factors must therefore be sought.

The differentiation of the three 'chronic' conditions is far from clear-cut. Disagreement exists over the significance of various bacteria recovered from the prostate and the 'cut-off' point regarding the number of white blood cells present in normal prostatic fluid. This is further aggravated by the use of the high-power field as a yardstick, not a standard counting chamber, in many publications.

Patients with abacterial prostatitis and prostatodynia are frequently resistant to standard treatments. In the abacterial prostatitis group several organisms have been implicated, including viruses, yeasts and chlamydia. The latter were thought to be the best candidate. However, in a recent study of such cases, biopsies of abnormal areas of the prostate, identified on ultrasound scan, confirmed a chronic inflammatory response in 86% but were unable to identify any evidence of persistent chlamydial infection. They were therefore unable to confirm the role of chlamydia as the infective agent in this group of patients (Doble *et al.*, 1989). A previous study from St Peter's Hospital reported that 61.3% of abacterial prostatitis cases studied had saprophytic organisms present in expressed prostatic secretion (EPS) compared with only 17.8% of normal controls, 26.1% of bacterial prostatitis and 31% of prostatodynia patients (Thin & Simmons, 1983). This raises the possibility that these Gram-positive organisms may play a part in the disease process. This possibility is controversial and there is considerable disagreement amongst authorities (Drach *et al.*, 1978).

The confirmation that a particular organism is pathogenic is extremely difficult in an area which is known to have a resident flora. This must, therefore, rest with the association of an inflammatory response to the presence of the organism concerned. It may take the form of an increase in leucocyte infiltration or a more specific immunological response to the organism. However, limitations of lower tract screening or the Stamey bacterial localization procedure are well known:

1 the EPS obtained does not represent the whole gland and prostatitis is thought to be a focal disease; and

2 there is always contamination from the urethra and associated glands.

In prostatitis, an increased number of organisms in the post-massage specimens associated with appropriate symptoms has been used to imply the causal role of the organism. There can be little doubt that in patients presenting with relapsing lower urinary tract infection, with normal upper tracts, the prostate is the commonest source of the infection (Meares & Stamey, 1968). This type of presentation in 'chronic prostatitis' is, however, felt to be uncommon (Mårdh and Colleen, 1975).

In normal controls, qualitative studies suggest that the flora of the normal prostate is varied and includes Gram-positive, Gram-negative and anaerobic organisms (Ambrose *et al.*, 1961; Murnaghan *et al.*, 1973; Mårdh & Colleen, 1975). These findings are supported by the culture of prostatic tissue taken at the time of surgery. Workers have found Gram-negative, Gram-positive and anaerobic organisms in surgical specimens from pain-free patients undergoing prostatic surgery for outflow obstruction and carcinoma — in 15 of 34 undergoing transurethral resection and three of three undergoing radical prostatectomy (Gorelick *et al.*, 1988). The use of qualitative culture techniques, however, prevents adjustment for urethral contamination, which is again inevitable. Quantitative culture, following a Stamey localization procedure, found almost no bacteria ($< 10^2$ colony forming units (cfu)/ml) in the voided bladder (VB2), EPS and VB3 of normal controls, but details of the types of organisms recovered were not given (Drach, 1974).

The pathogenic nature of the Gram-positive organisms, other than *Enterococcus faecalis*, is particularly uncertain. The absence of reported details of an associated inflammatory response (i.e. the number of leucocytes found in the EPS or VB3 in comparison with the VB1 and VB2) makes the assumption of the pathogenicity of these organisms based on the interpretation of quantitative culture results alone uncertain (Mårdh & Colleen, 1975). On the other hand, the *qualitative* culture of these saprophytic organisms, in the presence of a defined inflammatory response, again prevents confident analysis (Maged & Khafaga, 1965). However, agglutinins to staphylococci have been demonstrated in both the sera and the prostatic secretions in symptomatic patients (Maged & Khafaga, 1965) and clinical evidence of their pathogenic potential exists (Drach, 1974; Carson *et al.*, 1982).

Anatomical factors in prostatitis

Interest in the morphological anatomy of the prostate was stimulated by the apparent predisposition of Lowsley's posterior lobe to develop carcinoma. Other workers in the field have found a more widespread distribution of malignancy, but predominantly in the peripheral zone as described by McNeal (1968). A similar zonal distribution for inflammatory changes in the prostate was also found. On a histological basis, of 91 adult prostates removed at autopsy, 40 showed evidence of prostatitis. Twenty-four were confined to the peripheral zone, but only two involved the central zone alone. In those involving both, the changes in the central zone were usually less severe and often in continuity with the inflamed peripheral zone. This was thought to represent spill-over from the initial focus in the peripheral zone (McNeal, 1968).

Explanations for the zonal distribution of malignancy are based on the morphological differences of the parenchyma and proposed variations in their hormone sensitivity. In prostatitis, however, the regional variation can be better explained by anatomical and functional means.

Blacklock (1974) applied anatomical considerations in an attempt to explain the aetiology of bacterial prostatitis. Studying serially blocked normal prostates removed at post-mortem and prostates removed by total prostatectomy for prostatitis, he explained that the distribution of inflammatory lesions could be accounted for by ascending infection and certain anatomical factors (Blacklock, 1974). Bacterial prostatitis was felt to be a sexually acquired disease, being more common in married men and similar organisms being recovered from the introitus of their sexual partners. Anatomically, the alignment of the duct systems of each zone was felt to be of paramount importance. The ducts of the central zone are parallel with the ejaculatory ducts and both are in line with the lower prostatic urethra, aiding ejection from both down the urethra during intrinsic ejaculation. In the peripheral zone the ducts enter the urethra at 90° or more to the direction of flow. This alignment cannot aid in the propulsion of prostatic fluid down the urethra but was thought to produce turbulent mixing of the ejaculate. This turbulence and the spasmodic contraction of the uppermost fibres of the external urethral sphincter, during extrinsic ejaculation, were felt likely to result in the introduction of bacteria into the ducts of the peripheral zone.

Similarly, organisms in the prostatic urethra may be forced by high pressure into the prostate during micturition. This may result from failed relaxation of the external striated sphincter or distal obstruction, e.g. urethral stricture. The peripheral zone ducts are again more likely to reflux under pressure than those of the central zone, which may well be closed during periods of raised intraprostatic urethra pressure because of their angle of opening (Fig. 7.1).

Urethroprostatic reflux

Indirect proof of the intraprostatic reflux of urine was found by Sutor & Wooley (1974) during analysis of the constituents of prostatic calculi. They found 50% of prostatic calculi are formed, at least in part, by constituents derived from the urethral urine and not from the prostatic secretions. Subsequently, Meares (1980) in a review article concluded that reflux of infected urine into the prostatic ducts may be an important route of infection in cases of prostatitis.

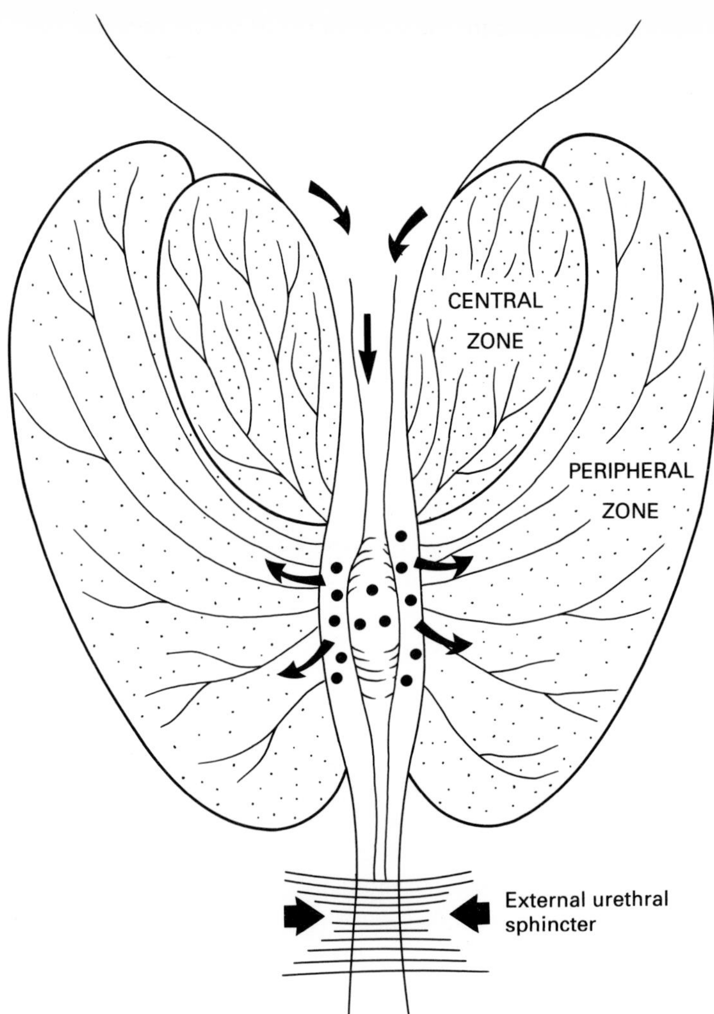

Fig. 7.1. The reflux of urine into the prostate.

Urethroprostatic reflux has subsequently been identified in paraplegics during voiding cystourethrography as a simple sign of abnormal function of the external urethral sphincter in this group of patients (Koyanagi *et al.*, 1982). Of the 15 patients identified in this series with high voiding pressures and failure to relax the sphincter during voiding, eight had persistent sphincter electromyographic activity during the void (somatic sphincter dyssynergia) but seven had silent electromyographic traces. Further investigation of the latter group revealed evidence of a sympathetic dyssynergia with an excessive increase in urethral pressure and catecholamine levels on changing from the lying to the sitting position. A moderate rise in the maximum urethral closure pressure (MUCP) is considered normal but the high voiding pressures found in the presence of a silent sphincter electromyography and a supersensitivity to alpha-adrenergic blockade suggest a sympathetic dyssynergia of the external urethral sphincter. In 12 of the

15 cases reflux was into the peripheral zone of the prostate. The central zone was only involved in four patients and always in the presence of reflux into the peripheral zone. This radiological evidence confirms the anatomical findings of Blacklock (1974) (Fig. 7.2).

A functional voiding disturbance?

Further confirmation of the presence of intraprostatic reflux was obtained using a suspension of carbon particles (Kirby *et al.*, 1982). In 10 male cadavers the instillation of a carbon particle suspension into the bladder until the intravesical pressure reached 50 cm of H_2O resulted in macroscopic evidence of reflux. From their illustrations it would again appear to be the peripheral zone that was involved. Similar findings occurred in seven of 10 cases undergoing transurethral prostatectomy for outflow obstruction. In five cases of abacterial prostatitis, confirmed by the analysis of the prostatic fluid, the bladder

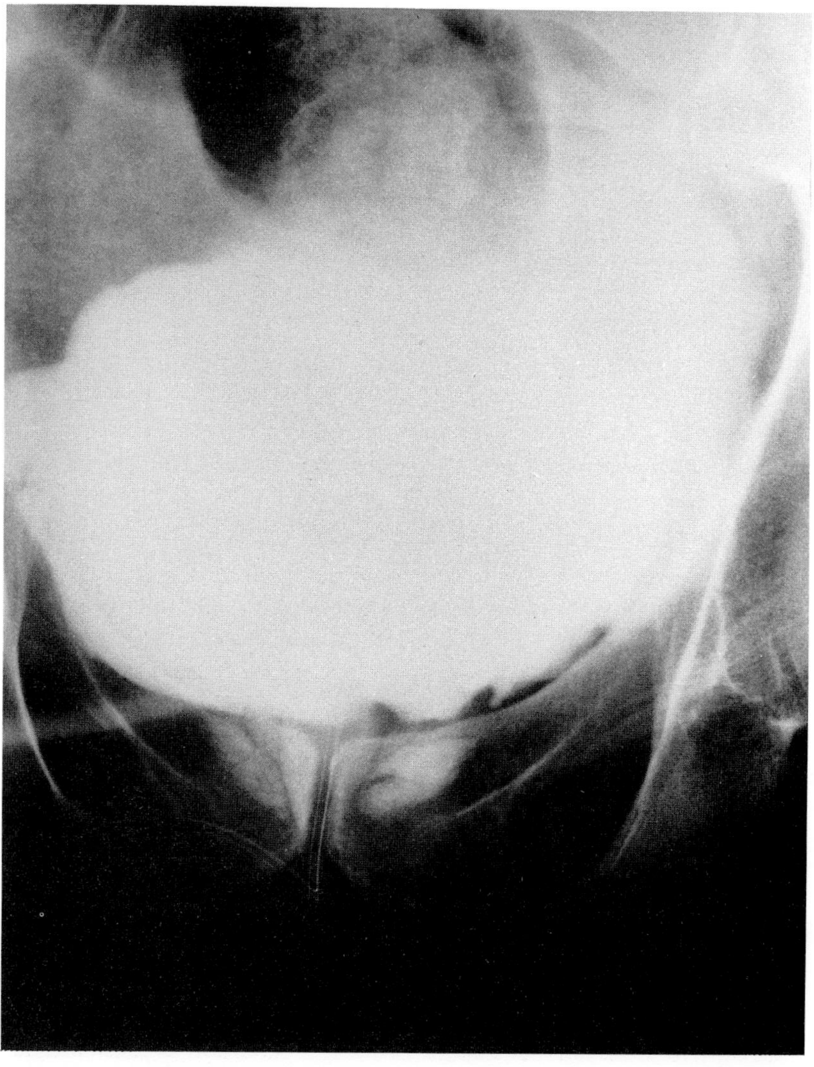

Fig. 7.2. Urethroprostatic reflux during videocystometry in a paraplegic.

was filled with a suspension of carbon particles by a urethral catheter. The patient was then asked to void and at 72 hours a prostatic massage was performed. In all cases numerous macrophages containing carbon particles were found in the expressed prostatic secretions. This work suggests that intraprostatic reflux is a common occurrence and the authors felt it was a significant factor in the development of abacterial prostatitis. However, 70% of those with outflow obstruction were also found to have intraprostatic reflux. Therefore, by itself reflux may not be sufficient to precipitate an inflammatory response.

In a retrospective review of 264 males referred for videocystometry, urethroprostatic reflux was identified in 11% of those investigated (Chapple *et al.*, 1990). The phase of the micturition cycle during which reflux was identified was investigated. In 27% this occurred during filling and was associated with unstable detrusor contractions and previous bladder-neck surgery. Reflux during voiding occurred in 50% of cases, seven had outflow obstruction, 10 were unstable, and three were normal. A 'stop test' precipitated reflux in a further seven patients (23%); all had bladder-neck obstruction. The incidence of symptoms suggestive of 'prostatitis' in this group was again low, supporting the findings of the previous authors but not their conclusions.

Blacklock (1986a) felt urinary reflux in small amounts into the prostate was probably a common occurrence and on its own was unlikely to be the cause for the initiation of an inflammatory response in the prostate. Other factors including the patient's local immunity, the contents of the urine, and the pressure of the reflux may all be important in subsequent development of an inflammatory response. In girls and women with dysfunctional voiding disturbances and recurrent urinary tract infections it has been suggested that raised intravesical pressure may result in ischaemic damage to the bladder mucosa resulting in an increased susceptibility to the invasion of Gram-negative organisms (Lapides & Diokno, 1970). This may also be the case in the prostatitis group of syndromes and the pressure of the urethroprostatic reflux may be significant.

Voiding abnormalities and the function of the external urethral sphincter in chronic prostatic pain

Patients with chronic prostatic pain often complain of a poor intermittent stream which is variable in nature. They often describe themselves as inhibited voiders, experiencing difficulty initiating voiding in 'public' toilets. These observations and the proposed aetiological significance of the reflux of urine into the prostate suggest an abnormality of external urethral sphincter function. In the normal initiation of voiding there is a synchronous and complete relaxation of the external urethral sphincter, as shown by a silent electromyographic trace, with the onset of the detrusor contraction. In fact, relaxation of the external urethral sphincter often occurs immediately prior to the onset of the detrusor contraction and may be an important initiating factor in normal micturition.

A functional voiding disturbance?

During an episode of acute bacterial prostatitis, typified by dysuria, frequency, haematuria and in some perineal pain, the flow rate has been shown to be reduced (Buck, 1975). A mean peak flow rate (PFR) of 17.14 ± 7.35 ml/s (mean ± SD) increased to 23.79 ± 6.20 ml/s following successful treatment ($P < 0.01$). The reduced peak flow was also associated with a slow rise to peak and a prolonged voiding time. Eradication of the infection also restored a normal voiding pattern. Electromyography (EMG) of the external urethral sphincter in the acute phase in four patients, using a needle electrode placed under digital rectal control, found a persistent low-grade interference pattern throughout voiding. This indicates a failure of the urethral sphincter to relax completely. These findings probably represent the normal response to painful micturition and in themselves cannot be implicated as an aetiological factor. In these circumstances, delayed eradication of infection from the urethra may result and urethroprostatic reflux may be precipitated. In the chronic 'prostatitis' group of patients, other than those presenting with relapsing urinary tract infection with positive mid-stream urine specimens, dysuria is often absent or minimal.

A prospective study of 27 patients with prostatodynia, confirmed by prostatic massage, found a similar reduction with a mean PFR of 16.2 ± 0.9 ml/s (Osborn *et al.*, 1981). Using the Brown & Wickham technique (Brown & Wickham, 1969), the mean maximum urethral closure pressure was found to be raised at 121 cm H_2O ± 9.23 SEM compared with documented controls. Psychological testing of these patients revealed an increased level of anxiety and the mean EMG voltage of the resting frontalis muscle was also raised. This suggested a generalized increase in striated muscle tone and symptomatic improvement was achieved in 50% with phenoxybenzamine (10 mg twice daily), and in 37% by baclofen (10 mg three times daily). The authors commented on the similarity of this group of patients with those suffering with the non-painful condition of the 'anxious bladder' (George & Slade, 1979). In the anxious bladder, typically the patients complained of daytime frequency, hesitancy, a poor stream and an inability to void in public toilets. Flow rates were again poor and often intermittent. Urodynamic studies in this group, performed in private, revealed weak poorly maintained detrusor contractions as the underlying cause, in the absence of clinical signs of neurological impairment. The authors also found an association with dyspepsia and anxiety disorders. A chronic sympathetically mediated systemic state was proposed to account for these findings in the anxious bladder.

Using rapid-fill gas cystometry with simultaneous perineal needle electromyography in 47 men with symptoms of dysuria, frequency, urgency, hesitancy and poor stream (22 with a diagnosis of 'chronic prostatitis'), Siroky *et al.* (1981) found three groups of voiding patterns. Firstly, 50% had bladder areflexia with non-relaxing pelvic floors, i.e. they were unable to initiate voiding under test circumstances. Secondly, 36% had detrusor hyperreflexia, and, thirdly, 14% were normal. Those in the first group often had a 'sawtooth' voiding pattern, the result of straining against a non-relaxed pelvic floor, similar to the intermittent stream of the 'anxious bladder' (George & Slade, 1979). Interestingly, of the 'normal' patients five had initial spasm of the pelvic floor musculature. Psychiatric and social disturbances were again common (55%) and five patients complained of urinary hesitancy in public. Treatment with diazepam resulted in symptomatic improvement in 15 of 18 with areflexic bladders and in three of five with initial spasm of the pelvic floor muscles. This improvement was again associated with a normalization of the flow pattern. In the reply to the editorial comments, the authors concluded that the areflexic pattern was manifested at times other than during the urodynamic tests and represented a true voiding abnormality, e.g. during voiding in public toilets.

During combined videocystometry and needle EMG of the external urethral sphincter in a further 20 cases of prostatodynia, 11 again failed to void (Barbalias *et al.*, 1983). In the nine who voided successfully synergistic voiding was described. The authors conclude from the nine (45%) who successfully voided, despite the test circumstances, that in prostatodynia the striated sphincter could not be implicated. However, as in the previous study 55% failed to initiate voiding under the test conditions, and voiding symptoms and flow patterns in this group of patients are well known to be variable, with patients describing good days and bad. In the non-voiders no comment is made on changes in sphincter activity or detrusor pressure during attempts to void. A more realistic conclusion would have been that 55% failed to initiate voiding, for an unknown reason, and the remaining 45% were synergistic voiders. Again, the mean maximum urethral closure pressure of the group was raised at 110 ± 6.88 cm H_2O compared with an age- and sex-matched control group mean of 60 ± 2.51 cm H_2O. This finding combined with electromyographic silence of the external sphincter during voiding, in some, suggested to the authors a sympathetically mediated dyssynergia as described by Awad & Downie (1977). In this series of 10 patients urethral constriction at the level of the external sphincter was improved by alpha-adrenergic blockade, suggesting a significant sympathetic component. All patients studied did, however, have clinically detectable neurological impairment, unlike the prostatodynia group reported by Barbalias *et al.* (1983).

The existence of a urethral supersensitivity to circulating catecholamines with an occult urethral neuropathy has been suggested in neurologically 'intact' patients to account for the exaggerated response to postural changes seen in some patients with voiding difficulties

(Parsons & Turton, 1980). In this paper the authors claimed that in normal individuals the urethral closure pressure does not change during alterations of posture. In a small group of patients with urethral obstruction, four female and one male, a rise of 11–88% (mean 41%) was found. Other authors have reported an increase ranging from 14 to 43% (mean 23%) on adopting the sitting position from lying in normal individuals (George & Feneley, 1979). Using a technique to mimic the circulatory changes of alterations in posture, by inflating pneumatic cuffs applied to both thighs, and by avoiding changes in spinal reflex activity, the changes in the maximum urethral closure pressure were reproduced (Parsons & Turton, 1980). This response was again reduced by 10 mg intravenous phentolamine, an alpha-adrenergic blocking agent. These findings support the role of a sympathetically mediated response to changes in posture in normal subjects. In some individuals this response appears to be abnormally increased and this can occur in the absence of overt neurological disease. This technique has not been applied to the 'prostatitis' group of patients.

The inability to void or voiding by abdominal straining in the absence of bladder-outflow obstruction appears common in the test circumstances in the prostatodynia group (Siroky *et al.*, 1981; Barbalias *et al.*, 1983). These patients also complain of difficulty initiating voiding in public toilets and this symptom, therefore, appears to be a genuine part of their voiding dysfunction. This failure of the 'micturition reflex' may result from damage to sacral or parasympathetic nerves or from idiopathic detrusor failure (Kirby *et al.*, 1983). In 28 patients such patients, 13 had no identifiable cause for their voiding difficulty. Two patients of this idiopathic group were found to have upper tract dilatation which was attributed to excessive abdominal straining. During filling cystometry a normal rise in the urethral pressure was found in the idiopathic group; this response was absent or reduced in those with a neurogenic lesion. In the neurogenic group the bladder neck was found to be open during filling and motor unit analysis of the external urethral sphincter revealed evidence of deinnervation and subsequent reinnervation, with increased duration and amplitude of the motor units. This was not the case in the idiopathic group and the cause for the loss of the micturition reflex in these patients was not determined. The authors speculated that the responsible factor was loss of corticopontine initiation of micturition, or failure of the detrusor muscle to respond to neural stimuli. The similarity of the voiding abnormality of this idiopathic group with those of the prostatodynia group and anxious bladder group cannot be avoided. Also, in two abdominal straining was sufficient to result in upper tract dilatation. This same situation could precipitate urethroprostatic reflux which may be important not only in the prostatodynia group of patients but also in those with prostatitis.

More recently, Meares (1986) described the urodynamic results of a further 64 cases of prostatodynia. His description was identical to those previously reported from his unit (Barbalias *et al.*, 1983) and was based on 35 patients who successfully voided. Importantly, 25% of this group had > 15 leucocytes/high powered field (hpf) on at least one occasion and would by many be described as suffering from non-bacterial prostatitis. Unfortunately, no distinction was made in the analysis of the results. The author did, however, comment that patients with non-bacterial prostatitis may also have an underlying voiding abnormality precipitating, by means of intraprostatic reflux, a chemical prostatitis.

The reduction of peak flow rates and voided volumes in acute prostatitis was also described by Blacklock (1986a). This was attributed to 'spasm' of the urethral sphincters, but invasive urodynamic studies were felt to be unethical under the circumstances of an active infection. Observation of the patients revealed spasm of the pelvic floor musculature, especially on standing. This may result in failure to eradicate infection from the prostate because of repeated urinary reflux and poor drainage of the inflamed prostatic ducts. The symptoms of spasm of these muscles, i.e. suprapubic, perineal, groin and testicular pain, are relieved by bed rest with an associated improvement in urinary flow parameters. No follow-up data are supplied and it is uncertain whether these findings are the result of the acute infection, and after successful treatment return to normal, or whether there is an underlying abnormality of the pelvic floor musculature resulting in a chronic voiding abnormality interrupted by occasional infected interludes. Certainly, 'pelvic floor tension myalgia' has many similarities with prostatodynia (Segura *et al.*, 1979). The syndrome is described in both men and women, and is characterized by continuous habitual contraction of the muscles of the pelvic floor. In the prostatodynia group increased frontalis muscle tension has been reported (Reading *et al.*, 1982) and this has led to speculation that the symptoms of prostatodynia are related to pelvic floor spasm as part of a generalized overactivity of the skeletal musculature (Blacklock, 1986b).

In a urodynamic study of 16 patients with prostatodynia, peak urinary flow rate was again reduced with a raised urethral closure pressure (Muhrer & Weidner, 1986). However, two patients were shown to have increased activity of the external urethral sphincter during voiding as recorded by electromyography; details of the technique used were not given. These patients were labelled as suffering from 'detrusor–sphincter dyssynergia' in the absence of any described neurological deficit. In these circumstances, it is more likely that the patient was suffering from a learnt functional voiding disorder, as occurs in children, with delayed relaxation of the external urethral sphincter after the onset of the detrusor contraction, rather than a true dyssynergic picture (Allen & Bright, 1978; Hinman, 1980; Koff, 1982). It has been proposed that in normal children this represents a transitional phase during toilet training whereby the child learns to prevent involuntary incontinence by forceful contraction of the

A functional voiding disturbance?

external urethral sphincter (Allen & Bright, 1978). In children with non-neurogenic or functional voiding disorders, successful long-term treatment has been achieved using a combination of bladder retraining and biofeedback (Maizels *et al.*, 1979; Hanson *et al.*, 1987; Hellström *et al.*, 1987; Keating & Cruz-Schmedel, 1988). A further patient, in this series, had increased involuntary electromyographic activity of the pelvic floor muscles as well as the external urethral sphincter, again suggesting a generalized increased tone of the striated muscles (see also Blacklock, 1986b).

The voiding abnormalities of prostatodynia have been attributed by several authors (see above) to abnormalities in the smooth muscle element of the sphincters resulting in poor flow rates and an increased urethral closure pressure. It has also been observed that many of the patients with prostatodynia have anal disorders which could be associated with an increased anal tone (Muhrer & Weidner, 1986). In a review of 75 patients with prostatodynia, only 12 had 'normal' proctological findings on examination. Haemorrhoids, proctitis and fissure in ano were the commonest visible abnormalities found, but 19 patients were described on rectal examination to have increased tone of the anal sphincter in the absence of any painful stimulus. Intraluminal manometry of the anal sphincter region, using a balloon catheter, in a number of patients revealed raised static pressures over a greater length of the anal canal.

Increased smooth muscle tone of both the anal canal and the bladder outlet was proposed as a common underlying cause for the anorectal abnormalities and voiding disorder found in prostatodynia patients.

George & Reading (1986) agreed that, whilst psychophysiological studies and urodynamic measurements in patients with prostatodynia or the 'anxious bladder' suggested the role of the sympathetic nervous system in these conditions, there was a lack of objective proof. The raised urethral closure pressure found in comparison to age-matched controls could equally be due to increased tone of the adrenergic smooth muscle, the external urethral sphincter, the periurethral striated muscle or a combination of these. It must also be remembered that the 'spasm' may be the result and not the cause of the perineal pain in the prostatodynia group. Similarly, in the anxious bladder a poor intermittent flow is associated with a low-amplitude poorly maintained detrusor contraction. This may be the result of chronic sympathetic stimulation suppressing the detrusor muscle whilst increasing the tone of the smooth muscle sphincters. Alternatively, over-inhibition of the micturition reflex as the result of chronic dysuria may occur. The loss of the micturition reflex has also been described in non-obstructive detrusor failure. In 28 patients, 9 male and 19 female, cauda equina lesions and pelvic nerve injuries accounted for 15, but in 13 patients no underlying neurological cause or autonomic dysfunction was identified (Kirby *et al.*, 1983). George & Reading concluded that, in the 'sensory' disorders of micturition, prostatodynia and the 'anxious bladder', no definite cause–effect relationship had been established between objective measures of sympathetic nervous system activity and the urodynamic findings. Similar findings could be explained by an as yet unidentified occult neuropathy or myopathy.

In 1987, Hellström *et al.* described three cases which they categorized as non-bacterial prostatitis but review of the clinical details reveals the absence of an inflammatory response in the post-massage specimens. These patients, who are best considered as suffering from prostatodynia, were investigated by videocystometry and simultaneous dynamic urethral pressure monitoring. In each, raised urethral pressures were described and in two spastic contraction–relaxation responses occurred in the urethra. In the second, the urodynamic trace reveals uncoordinated relaxation of the sphincters during voiding which can be attributed to the external urethral sphincter. In two cases the use of an S3 sacral root stimulator has resulted in symptomatic improvement. The authors attribute this to fatigue of the external sphincter which in its turn improves voiding and reduces urethroprostatic reflux.

The voiding abnormality in this group of conditions remains uncertain, particularly in those with true chronic prostatitis confirmed by the presence of excess leucocytes in the post-massage specimens. The function of the external striated sphincter during voiding has also not been fully established. The loss of the voiding reflex in many patients under test circumstances and the inhibited nature of the patients make investigation in a suitable environment essential to obtain reliable results.

Patients, materials and methods

At the Institute of Urology we have prospectively collected the results of those undergoing bacterial localization studies since October 1989. Eighty-five consecutive symptomatic patients were studied. Antibiotics were avoided for at least 5 days prior to prostatic massage. Quantitative culture techniques were employed and all positive cultures were identified by standard bacteriological techniques. Leucocyte counts were performed in a standard counting chamber. A diagnostic threshold of 500 white cells/mm^3 in the EPS and/or 40/mm^3 in the post-massage initial urine specimen (VB3) was used. Above this level the patient was assigned to the prostatitis group. Culture results were considered positive, i.e. attributable to the prostate, if organisms were recovered from the EPS and/or the VB3 with a 10-fold excess compared with the VB1 and VB2.

Secondly, 47 of these patients underwent synchronous medium-fill cystometry and concentric needle EMG of the external urethral sphincter. The needle was placed *in situ* under digital control. The needle was advanced towards the apex of the prostate until a good signal-to-noise ratio was obtained. Voiding was in the upright position in private to avoid inhibition.

Results

Using our diagnostic criteria, nine patients had abacterial prostatitis, 14 bacterial prostatitis and 53 prostatodynia. Nine patients were found to be suffering from urethritis with excess leucocytes being found in the initial specimen of urine (VB1). However, 30 patients with prostatodynia had positive cultures, i.e. bacteria were recovered from the post-massage specimens which could not be accounted for by urethral or bladder urine contamination, and in nine cases of 'bacterial prostatitis' the organisms were not widely accepted pathogens. Accepted urinary pathogens *E. coli* and *Enterococcus faecalis* were found in both the prostatitis and prostatodynia groups. Coagulase-negative staphylococci and coryneforms were recovered commonly and accounted for most pure cultures. Cultures were predominantly mixed (35 of 56 positive cultures) (Tables 7.1 & 7.2).

In those who underwent voiding studies five were excluded, two failed to void and three experienced marked dysuria during the test circumstances. Of the remaining 42, there were 31 with prostatodynia, three with abacterial prostatitis and eight with bacterial prostatitis. Symptoms of irritable bowel syndrome were present in 29% of patients, 50% described themselves as inhibited voiders and 26% had undergone

Table 7.1. Incidence of positive cultures in the post-massage specimens of the prostatitis group (19 screenings in 14 patients, cultures considered positive if the colony count in the VB3 or EPS is ×10 that of the VB1 and VB2, or the VB1 and VB2 are sterile)

Organism	No. of episodes (%)	No. of patients (%)
Enterococcus faecalis	5 (26)	5 (36)
Escherichia coli	1 (5)	1 (7)
Streptococcus milleri 3	1 (5)	1 (7)
Streptococcus sanguis	1 (5)	1 (7)
Non-haemolytic streptococci	1 (5)	1 (7)
Coagulase-negative staphylococci	8 (42)	6 (43)
Coryneforms	11 (58)	9 (64)
Bacteroides	1 (5)	1 (7)
Unidentified organism	2	2

Solitary organisms 5 (26%): *E. faecalis* 1
Coag.-neg. staph. 2
Diphtheroids 2

Table 7.2. Positive bacterial cultures in the post-massage specimens of the prostatodynia group (37 screenings in 30 patients, definition of positive culture as before)

Organism	No. of episodes (%)	No. of patients (%)
Enterococcus faecalis	10 (27)	7 (23)
Escherichia coli	3 (8)	3 (10)
Enterobacter agglomerans	1 (3)	1 (3)
Klebsiella	1 (3)	1 (3)
Acinetobacter	1 (3)	1 (3)
Group B *Streptococcus*	2 (5)	2 (7)
Alpha-haemolytic *Streptococcus*	6 (16)	6 (20)
Non-haemolytic *Streptococcus*	3 (8)	3 (10)
Non-specified *Streptococcus*	1 (3)	1 (3)
Coagulase-negative staphylococci	23 (62)	19 (63)
Staphylococcus aureus	1 (3)	1 (3)
Micrococcus	1 (3)	1 (3)
Coryneforms	15 (41)	15 (50)
Lactobacillus	1 (3)	1 (3)
Bacteroides	1 (3)	1 (3)
Anaerobic cocci	1 (3)	1 (3)
Mixed anaerobes	1 (3)	1 (3)
Unidentified organisms	2	2

Solitary organism 11 (30%): Coag.-neg. staph. 5
Diphtheroids 2
E. faecalis 1
E. coli 1
Alpha-haem. s. 1
Lactobacillus 1

previous bladder-outlet surgery. The mean PFR was 16.3 ml/s. Twenty-six were found to be asynchronous voiders with delayed relaxation of the external urethral sphincter from the onset of the detrusor contraction, as measured by persistent EMG activity (Fig. 7.3). All the abacterial prostatitis patients and five out of the eight with bacterial prostatitis had delayed relaxation of the external sphincter. The mean delay in relaxation was 26.6 s, but extended to 80 s, and was associated with a delayed onset of flow (mean 26 s), again measured from the start of the detrusor contraction. This delayed relaxation was associated with straining to initiate the flow, despite the onset of a detrusor contraction in 14 subjects. Mean maximum intravesical pressures during this period, until maximum flow had been achieved, was 99 cm H_2O measured from the symphysis pubis, in those who strained. In four other cases although synchronous 'bursts' of activity of the external urethral sphincter were identified during voiding. Six other cases had true bladder-outflow obstruction with raised voiding detrusor

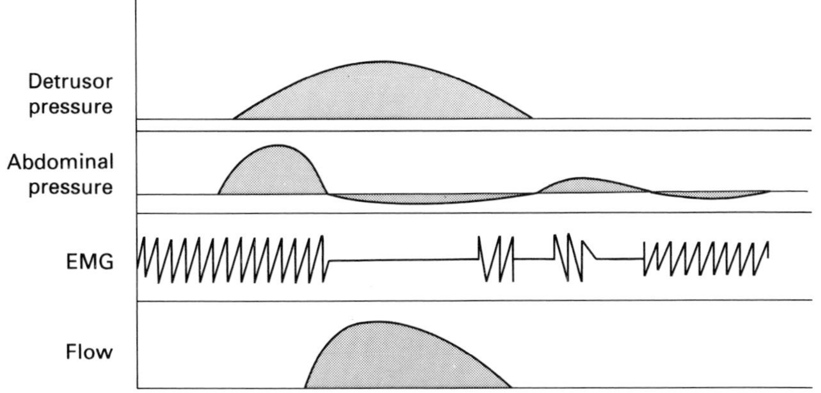

Fig. 7.3. Schematic representation of asynchronous voiding.

pressures and six had unstable detrusor contractions during bladder filling.

Discussion

Bacterial localization studies in chronic prostatic pain

Stamey localization studies are recommended for the investigation of patients suffering from chronic pain. Indeed the results are the main means of categorizing this diverse group of patients. There is considerable disagreement over the cut-off points to be used, i.e. the number of leucocytes in the post-massage specimens, and which bacteria are significant. The lack of suitable studies which combine both an inflammatory index and quantitative culture techniques prevents full assessment of this investigation, which is time-consuming, expensive and unpleasant for both the patient and the investigator. This lack of evidence is compounded by the poor response seen in patients treated by 'appropriate' antibiotic therapy.

In this study of 85 symptomatic patients, 53 were diagnosed to be suffering from 'prostatodynia'. However, 30 of this group had positive post-massage cultures which could not be accounted for by urethral contamination or infection of the bladder urine. The bacteria recovered included accepted urinary pathogens which occurred with the same frequency as seen in the 'prostatitis' group. The absence of an inflammatory response in the prostatodynia group suggests the organisms recovered were acting as commensals rather than pathogens. These findings are compatible with those previously reported from qualitative studies on the flora of the normal prostate (Ambrose *et al.*, 1961; Mårdh & Colleen, 1975; Gorelick *et al.*, 1988).

The flora of the anterior urethra is known to change frequently in the spinal injury group of patients and to be closely related to the perineal flora (Barnes *et al.*, 1992) and it is difficult to differentiate between colonization and contamination in this area. However, in two patients in the 'prostatodynia' group *Enterococcus faecalis* was recovered from the post-massage specimens on more than one occasion, each screening being separated by several weeks. From analysis of the colony counts this could not be explained by urethral or bladder urine contamination. This suggests true prostatic colonization in at least these two patients with accepted urinary pathogens. One patient had virtually no white blood cells present and the other an inadequate number to be considered a case of 'prostatitis' (Table 7.3). The distribution of bacteria attributed to the prostate between the prostatitis group and the prostatodynia group is dependent on the 'cut-off' point used in the diagnostic criteria. The level set in the prostatic secretions of 500 leucocytes/mm^3 was established by Simmons & Thin (1983) and is lower than that suggested by other authors (Drach *et al.*, 1978). However, using a higher limit would include more patients with urinary pathogens in the non-inflammatory group. Günthert (1986) during fertility studies has also found *E. coli* and enterococci in both the ejaculate and the prostatic fluid of otherwise asymptomatic patients.

Whichever level is chosen to divide the inflammatory condition prostatitis from the non-inflammatory condition prostatodynia it is merely an artificial 'all or nothing' cut-off. A better means of assessing the association of a particular organism with an inflammatory response is to compare the distribution of leucocytes in the groups with and without positive cultures for that organism in a statistical manner, as has been used to define significant bacteriuria. This has been done for the urinary pathogens, coagulase-negative staphylococci and diptheroids, both in the VB3 and the EPS. Using the Mann–Whitney two-tailed test there was no evidence of an association between the presence of any of these organisms and an increased number of leucocytes in the post-massage specimens. For the fastidious organisms coryneforms these findings mirror those reported by Gillespie and co-workers (1989) in the 'urethral syndrome'.

This suggests that factors other than the mere presence of a potential

Table 7.3. Two prostatodynia patients with persistent *E. faecalis* in the post-massage specimens (N.K., not known)

		Number of leucocytes in post-massage specimen	
		VB3	EPS
Patient 1	(a)	4	N.K.
	(b)	0	0
	(c)	4	0
Patient 2	(a)	10	150
	(b)	8	N.K.

pathogen are required to initiate an inflammatory response. Drach (1974) suggested that in chronic bacterial prostatitis there was an increased number of organisms recovered from the post-massage specimens compared with the normal subject who had almost no bacteria in the same specimens. He suggested bacterial prostatitis was likely if the VB1 and VB2 contained less than 3000 bacteria/ml and the EPS or VB3 contained more than 5000 bacteria/ml. However, Meares & Stamey (1972) stated that small numbers of organisms in chronic bacterial prostatitis were characteristic and significant, and urged follow-up of extremely small colony counts ($< 10^2$ organisms/ml).

We have further analysed our results combining together the colony counts into three groups: $< 10^4$ cfu/ml, 10^4-10^5 cfu/ml, and $> 10^5$ cfu/l. In our series, analysis of the inflammatory response, taking into consideration the colony count of coagulase-negative staphylococci, showed over 70% of screenings of each group had inadequate leucocytes present to be classified as suffering from prostatitis. Colony counts $> 10^5$ only occurred on two occasions in the VB3; both were associated with an absence of leucocytes. Colony counts of 10^4 or greater were not associated with a significant increase of inflammatory response compared with those $< 10^4$ (Mann–Whitney two-tailed test). This suggests that coagulase-negative staphylococci even in large numbers are not associated with 'prostatitis'.

Similarly, in this case of coryneforms, there was no evidence of a significant difference in the number of leucocytes, in the post-massage specimens, between those with $< 10^4$ colonies/ml and those with 10^4 or greater colonies/ml. This again suggests that increased numbers of coryneforms are not associated with an inflammatory response.

With regard to the urinary pathogens, mainly *E. faecalis* and *E. coli*, only one patient had $> 10^5$ organisms/ml in the prostatic secretions and this was associated with 8800 leucocytes/mm^3 in the same specimen. At the time of screening this patient had a significant bacteriuria with *E. coli*, but *E. faecalis* and bacteroids were also recovered from the post-massage specimens only. He had symptoms suggestive of a recurrent infective illness, with influenza-like symptoms and a high pyrexia associated with difficulty urinating. These subsided with antibiotic therapy but relapsed on withdrawal. He is the only patient in this series who falls into the 'chronic bacterial prostatitis' group described by Meares & Stamey (1968). This condition of a relapsing urinary tract infection attributed to an infective focus in the prostate has also been found to be rare by the other investigators (Mårdh & Colleen, 1975).

In the VB3, two of four screenings (50%) with 10^4 colonies or greater of a urinary pathogen fell into the 'prostatitis' group compared with only three of 16 (19%) with $< 10^4$ cfu/ml. This fact points to an association between an increased number of urinary pathogens and an increased number of leucocytes in the VB3. The numbers involved are small, however, and not statistically significant using the Mann–Whitney two-tailed test and association does not imply a causative role. A third factor may be responsible for both.

In light of these results, where urinary pathogens were also found in the absence of an inflammatory response on repeated screenings in the same subjects, factors other than the presence of the organism must be involved in the initiation of the 'disease process'. These factors may include autoimmune disease of the prostate, other epithelial-damaging conditions, e.g. high-pressure urinary reflux into the prostatic ducts, or an alteration of local immunity. In the then susceptible prostate opportunistic infection may occur.

Function of the external urethral sphincter in 'prostatitis'

Our results show an abnormality of external urethral sphincter EMG activity in 30 patients. Asynchronous relaxation of the sphincter occurring in 26, despite the onset of a detrusor contraction. This occurred in all groups studied and not just prostatodynia group. In the absence of an underlying neurological deficit the term detrusor sphincter dyssynergia should not be applied and these patients should be considered to be suffering from a functional voiding disorder as occurs in children. A similar pattern may, however, result from an occult neurological lesion. This asynchronous group of patients probably represents a failure in the development of the normal voiding reflex. A similar picture was described by Hellström *et al.* (1987) in three patients, but other workers in the field have failed to identify this abnormality and attributed their findings to the smooth muscle element of the urethra and bladder neck. In these series, failure to void was common and probably represented the complete loss of the voiding reflex under the test circumstances. Voiding was achieved in this series by careful attention to the patient's privacy, 50% of the patients describing themselves as lifelong inhibited voiders. Videocystometry was not attempted and, therefore, no comment of the function of the bladder neck can be made. The mean peak flow rate was 16.29 ml/s as reported by other workers. Only six patients were found to have raised voiding detrusor pressures suggesting true outflow obstruction and 11 of the patients had previously undergone bladder-outlet surgery in the form of a bladder-neck incision or transurethral resection of the prostate. Failure to completely relax the external sphincter was associated with poor-quality detrusor contractions.

Previous workers have suggested the role of urinary reflux in the aetiology of prostatitis, both bacterial and abacterial, and our findings would seem to add to this by proposing a functional obstructive element distal to the prostate. Straining during the initiation of voiding against a partially closed sphincter would promote reflux of urine under high pressure into the prostate. This may precipitate the onset of an inflammatory response with secondary bacterial infection occurring in those with bacterial prostatitis. In the abacterial group a chemical prostatitis or autoimmune disease has also been proposed. The painful symptoms in the prostatodynia group, who on prostatic massage reveal no evidence of an inflammatory response, is more difficult to explain. In this, the commonest category of the chronic painful prostate, the voiding abnormality found was identical to those with the inflammatory condition of prostatitis. The painful symptoms in all groups may arise from the pelvic floor, as proposed by Segura *et al.* (1979), rather than the prostate gland itself. Further evidence to support this theory is obtained in the apparent common asymptomatic nature of prostatitis as found by O'Shaughnessy *et al.* (1956) in army recruits and also those attending infertility clinics (Wolff *et al.*, 1991).

A functional voiding disturbance?

Conclusion

The bacterial flora of the prostate in the chronic painful prostate is varied and similar to that found in the normal prostate. Little evidence of an association could be found between the presence of these organisms and an inflammatory response. This includes accepted urinary pathogens which were found in the absence of an inflammatory response on repeated screening in two patients, suggesting true colonization of the prostate. The presence of these organisms alone does not seem sufficient to establish an inflammatory process; other factors must also be involved. The term chronic bacterial prostatitis should, therefore, be reserved for those few patients with recurrent urinary tract infections who respond to appropriate antibiotic therapy but relapse on withdrawal and have no other predisposing factors. In this group of patients localization studies have revealed the prostate as the source of the recurrent infection. This was the original description of chronic bacterial prostatitis (Meares & Stamey, 1968); the term has been extended in an attempt to explain the majority of patients with a benign painful prostate.

The asynchronous relaxation of the external sphincter during voiding in this group of patients would help to precipitate reflux of urine into the peripheral zone of the prostate. This was found in both the prostatitis and the prostatodynia groups of patients. However, reflux of urine by itself is probably a common occurrence. Straining to initiate micturition against a partially closed external urethral sphincter would result in the conduction of high pressure to the prostatic ducts. This high pressure may be important in causing epithelial damage, enabling bacterial invasion or implantation of 'foreign' materials, both resulting in an inflammatory response. However, the painful symptoms in the prostatodynia group, i.e. those with no identifiable inflammatory process, cannot easily be explained by these means and may arise from the pelvic floor itself. Further evidence that the inflammatory process identified by prostatic massage is not the cause for the painful symptoms is revealed by the common asymptomatic nature of the inflammatory changes. In 411 asymptomatic army recruits 38% were found to have an excess number of leucocytes present in the prostatic massage specimen on microscopy compared with 46% with symptoms suggestive of prostatitis. This finding prompted O'Shaughnessy *et al.* (1956) to ask the question 'Prostatitis — fact or fiction?'. Also, painless 'prostatitis' is commonly implicated in male infertility. The painful symptoms of 'prostatitis' may not therefore result from the 'inflammatory' process itself but from the functional voiding disorder or the patient's perception of the voiding disorder. This would explain the apparent success of stress therapy in this group of difficult patients (Miller, 1988).

References

Allen D.A. & Bright T.C. (1978) Urodynamic patterns in children with dysfunctional voiding problems. *J. Urol.*, **119**, 247–9.

Ambrose S.S., Taylor W.W. & Josefiak E.J. (1961) Flora of the male genitourinary tract. *J. Urol.*, **85**, 365–9.

Awad S.A. & Downie J.W. (1977) Sympathetic dyssynergia in the region of the external sphincter: a possible source of lower urinary tract obstruction. *J. Urol.*, **118**, 636–40.

Barbalias G.A., Meares E.M. & Sant G.R. (1983) Prostatodynia: Clinical and urodynamic characteristics. *J. Urol.*, **130**, 514–17.

Barnes D.G., Timoney A.G., Moulas G., Shaw P.J. & Sanderson P.J. (1992) Correlation of bacteriological flora of the urethra, glans and perineum with organisms causing urinary tract infection in the spinal injured male patient. *Paraplegia*, **30**, 851–4.

Blacklock N.J. (1974) Anatomical factors in prostatitis. *Br. J. Urol.*, **46**, 47–54.

Blacklock N.J. (1986a) Anatomic, urodynamic and other reasons for therapy failures in prostatitis. In: *Therapy of Prostatitis*, pp. 173–6. W. Zuckschwerdt Verlag, Munich.

Blacklock N.J. (1986b) Urodynamic and psychometric observations and their implications in the management of prostatodynia. In: *Therapy of Prostatitis*, pp. 201–6. W. Zuckschwerdt Verlag, Munich.

Brown M. & Wickham J.E.A. (1969) The urethral pressure profile. *Br. J. Urol.*, **41**, 211–17.

Buck A.C. (1975) Disorders of micturition in bacterial prostatitis. *Proc. Roy. Soc. Med.*, **68**, 508–11.

Carson C.C., McGraw V.D. & Zwadyk P. (1982) Bacterial prostatitis caused by *Staphylococcus saprophyticus*. *Urology*, **19**, 576–8.

Chapple C.R., Blease S.C.P. & Rickards D. (1990) What is the clinical significance of urethroprostatic reflux as a radiological finding during videocystourethrography in neurologically normal patients? *Eur. Urol.*, **17**, 296–8.

Doble A., Thomas B.J., Walker M.M., Harris J.R., Witherow R.O., Taylor & Robinson D. (1989) The role of chlamydia trachomatis in chronic abacterial prostatitis: A study using ultrasound guided biopsy. *J. Urol.*, **141**, 332–3.

Drach G.W. (1974) Problems in diagnosis of bacterial prostatitis: gram-negative, gram-positive and mixed infections. *J. Urol.*, **111**, 630–6.

Drach G.W., Fair W.R., Meares E.M. & Stamey T.A. (1978) Classification of the benign diseases associated with prostatic pain: prostatitis or prostatodynia? *J. Urol.*, **120**, 266.

George N.J.R. & Feneley R.C.L. (1978) The importance of postural influences on urethral musculature. Proceedings of the VIII International Continence Society Meeting, Manchester, 117–18.

George N.J.R. & Reading C. (1986) Sympathetic nervous system and the dysfunction of the lower urinary tract. *Clinical Science*, **70** (Suppl. 14), S69–S76.

George N.J.R. & Slade N. (1979) Hesitancy and poor stream in younger men without outflow tract obstruction — the anxious bladder. *Br. J. Urol.*, **51**, 506–9.

Gillespie W.A., Henderson E.P., Linton K.B. & Smith P.J. (1989) Microbiology of the urethral (frequency and dysuria) syndrome. A controlled study with 5-year review. *Br. J. Urol.*, **64**, 270–4.

Gorelick J.I., Senterfit L.B. & Darracott Vaughan E. Jr. (1988) Quantitative bacterial tissue cultures from 209 prostatectomy specimens: Findings and implications. *J. Urol.*, **139**, 57–60.

Hanson E., Helström A.-L. and Hjälmås K. (1987) Non-neurogenic discoordinated voiding in children. The long-term effect of bladder retraining. *Z. Kinderchir.*, **42**, 109–11.

Hellström A.-L., Hjälmås K. & Jodal U. (1987) Rehabilitation of the dysfunctional bladder in children: Method and 3-year followup. *J. Urol.*, **138**, 847–9.

Hellström W.J.G., Schmidt R.A., Lue T.F. & Tanagho E.A. (1987) Neuromuscular dysfunction in nonbacterial prostatitis. *Urology*, **30**, 183–8.

Hinman F. Jr. (1980) Syndromes of vesical incoordination. In: *Urologic Clinics of North America*, Vol. 7, No. 2, pp. 311–19. Saunders, Philadelphia.

Keating J.C. & Cruz-Schmedel D. (1988) Urodynamic feedback therapies for retentive dysfunctions. *J. Manip. Physiol. Ther.*, **11**, 190–4.

Kirby R.S., Lowe D., Bultitude M.I. & Shuttleworth K.E. (1982) Intra-prostatic urinary reflux: an aetiological factor in abacterial prostatitis. *Br. J. Urol.*, **54**, 729–31.

Kirby R.S., Fowler C., Gilpin S.-A., Holly E., Milroy E.J., Gosling J.A. & Bannister R. (1983) Non-obstructive detrusor failure. A urodynamic, electromyographic, neurohistochemical and autonomic study. *Br. J. Urol.*, **55**, 653–9.

Koff S.A. (1982) Bladder-sphincter dysfunction in childhood. *Urology*, **19**, 457–61.

Koyanagi T., Arikado K., Takamatsu T. & Tsuji I. (1982) Prostatic reflux: A simple radiographic sign in recognising dysfunctioned voiding from external sphincter disorders. *J. Urol.*, **128**, 93–7.

Lapides J. & Diokno A.C. (1970) Persistence of the infant bladder as a cause for urinary infection in girls. *J. Urol.*, **103**, 243–8.

McNeal J.E. (1968) Regional morphology and pathology of the prostate. *Amer. J. Clin. Path.*, **49**, 347–57.

Maged Z. & Khafaga H. (1965) Bacteriological and serological study of chronic prostatitis patients. *Br. J. Vener. Dis.*, **41**, 202–7.

Maizels M., King L.R. & Firlit C.F. (1979) Urodynamic biofeedback: A new approach to treat vesical sphincter dyssynergia. *J. Urol.*, **122**, 205–9.

Mårdh P.-A. and Colleen S. (1975) Search for uro-genital tract infections in patients with symptoms of prostatitis. *Scand. J. Urol. Nephrol.*, **9**, 8–16.

Meares E.M. (1977) Serum antibody titres in urethritis and chronic bacterial prostatitis. *Urology*, **10**, 305–9.

Meares E.M. (1980) Prostatitis syndromes: New perspectives about old woes. *J. Urol.*, **123**, 141–7.

Meares E.M. (1986) Prostatodynia: Clinical findings and rationale for treatment. In: *Therapy of Prostatitis*, pp. 207–12. W. Zuckschwerdt Verlag, Munich.

Meares E.M. & Stamey T.A. (1968) Bacterial localisation patterns in bacterial prostatitis and urethritis. *Invest. Urol.*, **5**, 492–518.

Meares E.M. & Stamey T.A. (1972) The diagnosis and management of bacterial prostatitis. *Br. J. Urol.*, **44**, 175–9.

Miller H.C. (1988) Stress prostatitis. *Urology*, **32**, 507–10.

Muhrer K.H. & Weidner W. (1986) Proctological aspects of pelvic disorders in patients with prostatodynia. In: *Therapy of Prostatitis*, pp. 213–17. W. Zuckschwerdt Verlag, Munich.

Murnaghan G.F., Tynan A.P., Farnsworth R.H. & Harvey K. (1974) Chronic prostatitis — An Australian view. *Br. J. Urol.*, **46**, 55–9.

Osborn D.E., George N.J.R., Rao P.N., Barnard R.J., Reading C., Marklow C. & Blacklock N.J. (1981) Prostatodynia — physiological characteristics and rational management with muscle relaxants. *Br. J. Urol.*, **53**, 621–3.

O'Shaughnessy E.J., Parrino P.S. & White J.D. (1956) Chronic prostatitis — fact or fiction? *JAMA*, **160**, 540–2.

Parsons K.F. & Turton M.B. (1980) Urethral supersensitivity and occult urethral neuropathy. *Br. J. Urol.*, **52**, 131–7.

Reading C., Osborn D.E., George N.J.R., Marklow C. & Blacklock N.J. (1982) Prostatodynia, a preliminary psychophysiological investigation. *Bio. Psychol.*, **15**, 283.

Segura J.W., Joachim L.O. & Greene L.F. (1979) Prostatosis, prostatitis or pelvic floor tension myalgia? *J. Urol.*, **122**, 168–9.

Shortliffe L.M., Wehner N. & Stamey T.A. (1981) The detection of a local prostatic immunologic response to bacterial prostatitis. *J. Urol.*, **125**, 509–15.

Simmons P.D. & Thin R.N. (1983) A method for recognising non-bacterial prostatitis: Preliminary observations. *Br. J. Vener. Dis.*, **59**, 306–10.

Siroky M.B., Goldstein I. & Krane R.J. (1981) Functional voiding disorders in men. *J. Urol.*, **126**, 200–4.

Stamey T.A., Meares E.M. & Winningham D.G. (1970) Chronic bacterial prostatitis and the diffusion of drugs into the prostatic fluid. *J. Urol.*, **103**, 187–94.

Sutor D.J. & Wooley S.E. (1974) The crystalline composition of prostatic calculi. *Br. J. Urol.*, **46**, 533–5.

Thin R.N. & Simmons P.D. (1983) Chronic bacterial and non-bacterial prostatitis. *Br. J. Urol.*, **55**, 513–18.

Wolff H., Bezold G., Zebhauser M. & Meurer M. (1991) Impact of clinically silent inflammation on male genital tract organs as reflected by biochemical markers in semen. *J. Androl.*, **12**, 331–4.

Young H.H. & Davies D.M. (1926) Urogenital infections and infestations: General. In: *Practice of Urology*, Vol. II, pp. 160–6 & 196–212. Saunders, Philadelphia.

8 Advances in the treatment of chronic prostatitis

T.K. SHAH

Introduction

Several important advances have been made in the last two to three decades in resolving the problems associated with this very common condition: firstly, in appreciating that this is not a single entity but rather a group of syndromes conveniently grouped under a common label of chronic prostatitis because of their similar clinical presentations; secondly, that these syndromes may have quite different pathogenesis and aetiological factors; and, finally, significant progress has been made in exploring newer techniques and drugs to find more effective and lasting cures in the management of these syndromes. Despite these efforts chronic prostatitis still remains an enigma in some respects. It is a condition which is a constant and recurring source of distress to the patient and a frustrating condition to treat for the clinician.

Sometimes labelled as prostatitis syndrome, it is in fact a group which encompasses three different entities: chronic bacterial prostatitis; chronic abacterial prostatitis; and prostatodynia. In spite of extensive research by dedicated workers, the controversy over the aetiology and pathogenesis of the condition remains unresolved to a great degree (Orland *et al.*, 1985). What is not quite explained is whether these three entities are various stages in the same disease process or are distinct diseases in their own rights not necessarily connected to each other. The evidence so far seems to indicate that the latter is more likely to be the case. Several factors may be responsible in the aetiology and pathogenesis which are apparently different for the three conditions.

Investigation

These three entities are clinically difficult if not impossible to differentiate. The distinction is, therefore, based primarily on microscopic and bacteriological findings of the fractionated urine specimen and prostatic expressate as described by Meares & Stamey (1968). The findings on the video-urodynamic studies may, however, substantiate the diagnosis of prostatodynia (Barbalias *et al.*, 1983) and may help differentiate it from chronic abacterial prostatitis and other conditions which may mimic it very closely such as pelvic floor myalgia, adductor muscle strain, chronic traumatic osteitis pubis, and detrusor–sphincter dyssynergia (Sinaki *et al.*, 1977; Segura *et al.*, 1979; Siroki *et al.*, 1981). Furthermore investigations with X-rays and electromyography may be required for the differential diagnosis.

As the three types of chronic prostatitis have different causes and different findings on investigations, the management strategies described for the three also differ. Each of them in turn presents with a substantial treatment challenge. The conventional treatments produce little relief if any and relapses are common. The difficulty in their management is apparent from the astronomical list of therapies described in the literature. For the treatment to produce benefit it is, therefore, important to comprehensively investigate and establish the diagnosis before initiating any therapy.

Management

With minor differences the three syndromes of chronic prostatitis present with a fairly common symptom complex. There is usually a variety of irritative lower urinary tract symptoms with dysuria, urgency, frequency, and nocturia. Pain, however, is the predominant symptom and is present around the genitalia and the pelvic area. Post-ejaculatory pain may be the most prominent symptom. In fact all the symptoms may be precipitated following intercourse. Classically the disease has a waxing and waning course. The patients may generally feel very unwell with malaise during a flare-up. Chronic bacterial prostatitis patients may give a previous history of urinary tract infection, while the patients with prostatodynia may have very little in terms of voiding disturbance but a strong history of pain. Physical examination may reveal no significant abnormality.

Not many would disagree that chronic prostatitis is one of the most difficult conditions to treat in urology. It is mostly refractory to the conventional treatments, such as antibiotics, alpha-adrenergic blockers, non-steroidal anti-inflammatory drugs, and other empirical manoeuvres. The response to these therapies is poor and relapse rate is high (Meares & Barbalias, 1983). Considerable work has gone into finding newer drugs and techniques in the management of these syndromes. A new therapy recently described is deep localized microwave hyperthermia.

The beneficial effects of heat for the relief of pain in chronic prostatitis has been well known to men. Many interesting methods have been described over the years for the delivery of heat to the prostate, e.g. hot sitz baths and warm compresses. All of these depend on conduction of heat energy from the source to the depths of the prostate; hence predictably none proved to be entirely satisfactory. In contrast, the microwaves are delivered by radiation of the energy from the source to the target. The microwave-emitting probe is placed in close proximity to the prostate, either in the rectum or in the prostatic urethra, producing hyperthermia by concentrating the radiated energy on the prostate.

In a pilot study at the Institute of Urology, London using microwave hyperthermia we have treated 50 patients with chronic prostatitis over a period of 2 years. In a second study which was designed to be randomized and double-blind with placebo control we have treated a further 30 patients.

In the pilot study patients with all three types of chronic prostatitis, i.e. chronic bacterial prostatitis, chronic abacterial prostatitis, and prostatodynia, were included. Three different types of machines were used to deliver the microwaves using both the transurethral and transrectal route. The results of this pilot study have been very encouraging in chronic abacterial prostatitis and prostatodynia but not in chronic bacterial prostatitis. However, the need for a placebo-controlled trial to demonstrate the efficacy of this form of treatment was greatly felt.

We have since undertaken a double-blind placebo-controlled trial using the transrectal approach to induce hyperthermia in patients with chronic abacterial prostatitis and prostatodynia. The early results of this trial confirm the findings of the pilot study. Though there is a placebo effect, the beneficial effects obtained by the active treatment are significantly higher. Moreover, we have seen from our pilot study that the beneficial effects of this form of treatment can be sustained for long periods.

Chronic bacterial prostatitis

Chronic bacterial prostatitis is classified and differentiated upon the finding of inflammatory cells and positive culture of the expressed prostatic secretion and post-massage urine specimen (VB3).

This form of prostatitis should logically be easy to treat with appropriate antibiotics. Unfortunately, this is not so simple. The anti-bacterial treatment is complicated by the factors governing the diffusion and concentration of drugs across the prostatic epithelial membrane from the plasma into the prostatic fluid. Stamey and associates (Winningham & Stamey, 1968; Stamey *et al.*, 1970) showed that factors like the lipid solubility of the drug, the degree of ionization in the plasma, and the protein binding of the drug govern the degree of diffusion, while the pH gradient across the epithelial membrane and the dissociation characteristics, i.e. acidic or basic nature of the antibiotic, determine its concentration in the prostate. Many other studies on chronic bacterial prostatitis in the last two decades have also helped us improve our understanding of this condition and the difficulties associated with its treatment such as the specific immunological factors and other non-specific host defences like the prostatic anti-bacterial factor (Fair *et al.*, 1976). Considering the nature of chronic bacterial prostatitis and the difficulties associated with getting the effective antibiotic in sufficient concentration to eradicate the bacteria it is not surprising that even the best available antibiotic will not cure every patient. Recent clinical studies suggest that the quinolones which are active against most of the bacteria responsible for chronic bacterial prostatitis are perhaps the most effective antibacterial agents, but these should be prescribed at an early stage and for long periods to produce the best results (Kumamoto *et al.*, 1987; Ball, 1989; Ikeuchi, 1990; Morikawa *et al.*, 1990; Aagaard & Madsen, 1991). Trimethoprim alone and sulphamethoxazole–trimethoprim combination and the role of some of the newer tetracyclines (minocycline, doxycycline) have also been studied quite extensively, their effectiveness closely follow the fluoroquinolones (Meares, 1973, 1975; Paulson & White, 1978; Paulson *et al.*, 1986; Szolnoki & Keri, 1989; Ikeuchi, 1990). To produce high concentrations of antibiotics in the prostate innovative techniques have been described such as transrectal intraprostatic injection of gentamicin (Baert *et al.*, 1983), transperineal injections of amikacin or tobramycin under ultrasound control into the echogenic zone or into the external prostate gland (Jimenez-Cruz *et al.*, 1988), anal submucosal injections of gentamicin (Shafik, 1991), and trapping the antibiotics in the prostatic urethra by specially designed catheters with balloons blocking the drug from passing into either the bladder or the membranous urethra and instilling the antibiotic directly into this enclosed posterior urethra (Cheng & Huang, 1987). Results of all these methods show a good clinical response and appear quite useful in a difficult condition; however, more clinical trials are required before such therapies are established.

One of the reasons for the failure of antibiotic therapy and the recurrence of symptoms in chronic bacterial prostatitis is the presence of infected prostatic calculi (Ey Kyn *et al.*, 1974). The bacteria are locked inside the calculi which cannot be sterilized by antibiotics. Surgically removing all the infected calculi and the prostatic tissue may be the only effective way of curing the disease. Indeed, before the advent of effective antibiotics for treatment of chronic bacterial prostatitis, the only alternative for patients who failed conventional treatment was surgical removal of the gland. High cure rates with transurethral resection of hyperplastic prostatic tissue (TURP) have been claimed by some workers (Smart & Jenkins, 1973; Smart *et al.*, 1976) but is generally agreed by most to be around 33% (Orland *et al.*, 1985). The reasons for these poor results are obvious, since it has been shown that the focus of infection in chronic bacterial prostatitis is more commonly found in the peripheral part of the gland rather than in the central part (McNeal, 1972; Doble & Carter, 1989) and since in both TURP and retropubic prostatectomy the peripheral glands are not removed the infected foci persist. The only sure cure would be a total prostatectomy but the complications and the risks of such an operation eclipse the benefits.

Chronic abacterial prostatitis

Chronic abacterial prostatitis is characterized by the presence of increased numbers of inflammatory cells in the prostatic expressates and post-massage urine specimen (VB3). However, on culture these specimens are sterile. The abnormally high number of leucocytes on Stamey's screen in chronic abacterial prostatitis indicates the inflammatory nature of this condition; however, no infectious cause has been demonstrated in spite of quite extensive search by several workers (Meares, 1980; Berger *et al.*, 1989). Hence, treatment using antimicrobial agents is ineffective and unwarranted (Meares, 1987, 1983). If infection with *Chlamydia* or *Ureaplasma* is suspected a short course of tetracyclines is justified and may be effective. In most of the patients, for lack of any specific treatment, clinicians usually end up prescribing short courses of antibiotics. Thin & Simmons (1983) have shown that tetracyclines (minocycline) can reduce the leucocyte count in the prostatic expressate. Trimethoprim was shown to be less effective in this respect and co-trimoxazole or diazepam had poor results. The poor results with co-trimoxazole were attributed to an insufficient amount of trimethoprim in the combination. In the same study the best symptomatic response was, however, seen with trimethoprim followed by diazepam and then by minocycline. Co-trimoxazole had the poorest clinical response. Generally, for want of evidence of any specific aetiology, the treatment is mostly empirical and is aimed at relieving the symptoms only. During the flare-up brief courses of alpha-adrenergic blockade and non-steroidal anti-inflammatory drugs may help in relieving the symptoms. Other treatments suggested are the liberal use of hot sitz bath, prostatic massage, antihistamines, benzodiazepines and anticholinergics (Meares, 1980; Orland *et al.*, 1985; Ogawa *et al.*, 1989). Treatment with pollen extracts, cernilton (Buck *et al.*, 1989), surfactant, Pantosan polysulphate sodium (Wedren, 1987, 1989) and oestrogens (Nelson, 1952; Mackenzie, 1986) has also shown significant improvement in symptoms. Stress prostatitis is the term suggested by Miller (1988) for patients with non-bacterial prostatitis or prostatodynia. He has recommended stress therapy alone in the management of these patients. However, larger series with controlled trials are needed for establishing these forms of therapies.

Prostatodynia

The aetiology and pathogenesis of prostatodynia are even more ill-understood and consequently the treatment is comparatively more disappointing. The disease is diagnosed on sterile cultures and absence of inflammatory cells in all specimens on Stamey's screen. Several workers have shown a voiding abnormality in patients with prostatodynia on video-urodynamic studies (Barbalias *et al.*; 1983; Meares, 1987, 1991; Barbalias, 1990; Barnes *et al.*, 1991a). This consists of reduction in both average and peak flow rates, an increase in maximum urethral closing pressure, incomplete funnelling of the bladder neck and narrowing at the level of the striated sphincter. Barbalias (1990) has, however, demonstrated the same pattern in non-prostatodynia patients and concludes that these changes may be only a step in a chain of events leading finally to chronic non-specific prostatitis, Whatever the sequence of happenings in this functional disorder, treatment with alpha-adrenergic-blocking drugs produces relief in the symptoms and improvement in the voiding disorder in some patients (Meares, 1980; Osborn *et al.*, 1981; Orland *et al.*, 1985). Stress and psychosomatic causes have been highlighted by some workers and treatment aimed at stress relief and psychiatric counselling has met with some success (Miller, 1988; Krieger & Egan, 1991).

Treatment of chronic prostatitis in general has met with disappointment. Patients who may show initial improvement do not maintain their remission for very long and relapses are seen commonly. This has certainly prompted numerous workers all around the world to research into newer techniques and ideas to treat this common condition.

Microwave hyperthermia in the treatment of chronic prostatitis

Since the initial work by Yerushalmi (1988) and Servadio *et al.*, (1987) several clinical series have now been reported in the literature on deep microwave hyperthermia of the prostate in the treatment of benign hyperplasia, using both transrectal and transurethral routes. The results generally show a 60–70% subjective improvement in the symptoms. Although the objective improvement in the flow rates, residual volumes, and the prostatic size are not as impressive, especially when compared with the transurethral resection of the prostate, the progress is significant and the complication rate minimal. Servadio *et al.* (1986, 1987) first reported the use of microwave hyperthermia in the treatment of chronic abacterial prostatitis using a skirt-type transrectal antenna to raise the temperature to 42.5°C (± 1°C) with marked improvement in the symptoms. Barnes *et al.* (1991a) reported the results of a pilot study on the treatment of benign prostatic pain in 11 patients. The results of this work were quite encouraging. This prompted us to utilize this method of treatment in a larger group.

The pilot study

Patients and method

- Fifty patients with chronic prostatic pain of benign prostatic origin were treated with microwave hyperthermia.
- All patients had had symptoms for prolonged periods and had failed to respond to conventional treatments.

• All had sought alternate treatments.
• All patients were scored according to the intensity of their symptoms on a specially designed scorecard.
• Specific investigations prior to the treatment included serum PSA; Stamey's screen; transrectal ultrasound; and ultrasound-guided prostate biopsy of suspicious areas.
• Patients were grouped according to the findings of the Stamey's screen into chronic bacterial prostatitis (5 patients), chronic abacterial prostatitis (12 patients), and prostatodynia (33 patients).

Three different microwave machines were employed

1 A Primus machine by Technomatix (33 patients) which uses a 915 MHz microwave generator with a transrectal probe and a water-cooling system for the rectal mucosa. Intraprostatic temperatures are estimated by the machine (and vary directly with the input power); a urethral catheter is not required.
2 A Thermex 11 by Direx which uses a transurethral heating electrode which is part of a modified Foley's catheter. The temperature is recorded by a thermocouple placed adjacent to the heating electrode and is considered the maximum treatment temperature.
3 A Prostathermer by Biodan Medical, which heats the prostate by a transrectal applicator with a microwave emission of 915 MHz. There is a cooling system for the rectal wall and a urethral catheter is placed to monitor the temperature in the prostatic urethra.

Treatment schedules

Note that all treatments were on an outpatient basis.

Primus
• Four to six 1-hour treatments spread over 3–6 weeks.
• Treatments in supine position.
• No analgesia or anaesthesia required.
• Maximum temperatures between 43 and 44°C.

Thermex 11
• Single session of 2–3 hour duration.
• Treatments in supine or sitting position.
• 1% lignocaine jelly per urethra 10 minutes before urethral catheterization.
• Gentle traction on the catheter after inflation of the intravesical balloon to fix the heating unit in the prostatic urethra.
• Maximum temperature between 42 and 45°C.

Prostathermer
• Six 1 hour treatments at weekly intervals.
• Treatments in supine or semi-lithotomy position.
• 1% lignocaine jelly per urethra before urethral catheterization.
• Maximum temperature between 42 and 43°C.

Follow-up

Post-treatment, patients were followed up at 6 weeks, 3 months, 6 months, and then at yearly intervals. The longest follow-ups are over 2 years. At the follow-up, symptoms were scored again. Less then 50% improvement in the score was considered a treatment failure or relapse.

Results of the pilot study

The results from our pilot study show a useful response in the symptoms of a significant number of patients with chronic prostatic pain who had failed to respond to conventional treatments. However, the response in the chronic bacterial prostatitis group was very poor, in fact no patient showed any improvement at 3 months in this group. The results are shown in Tables 8.1–8.4.

- 68% of the 50 patients in the whole group showed significant subjective improvement at 6 weeks post-treatment.
- Most of the patients who showed improvement continued to maintain the improvement with a slow relapse rate.

Table 8.1. Pilot study: results of patients with chronic prostatitis (CP)

Follow-up	Total no. patients	> 50% Improvement		< 50% Improvement or relapse	
		No.	%	No.	%
6 weeks	50	34	68	16	32
3 months	34	29	85	5	15
6 months	29	25	86	4	14
1 year	24	18	75	6	25
2 years	14	11	79	3	21

Table 8.2. Pilot study: results of patients with chronic bacterial prostatitis (CBP)

Follow-up	Total no patients	> 50% Improvement		< 50% Improvement or relapse	
		No.	%	No.	%
6 weeks	5	1	20	4	80
3 months	1	0	0	1	100
6 months					
1 year					
2 years					

Table 8.3. Pilot study: results of patients with chronic abacterial prostatitis (CAP)

		> 50% Improvement		< 50% Improvement or relapse	
Follow-up	Total no. patients	No.	%	No.	%
6 weeks	12	10	83	2	17
3 months	10	8	80	2	20
6 months	8	7	87	1	14
1 year	7	5	71	2	33
2 years	5	4	80	1	25

Table 8.4. Pilot study: results of patients with prostatodynia (PD)

		> 50% Improvement		< 50% Improvement or relapse	
Follow-up	Total no. patients	No.	%	No.	%
6 weeks	33	23	70	10	30
3 months	23	21	91	2	9
6 months	21	18	86	3	14
1 year	17	13	76	4	14
2 years	9	7	78	2	22

- At 2 years 14 patients were available for evaluation with 11 patients (79%) continuing to maintain their initial improvement.
- Best subjective improvement was seen in the chronic abacterial prostatitis group followed by the prostatodynia group. Chronic bacterial prostatitis patients had the poorest response and all relapsed at 3 months.

Although the Prostathermer showed the best percentage improvement there were too few patients in this group to make the difference significant. The relapse rate with the three machines was approximately the same.

Minimal discomfort was experienced during the treatment. Primus was perhaps tolerated best since there was no urethral catheterization. Operator and patient convenience was best with the Thermex 11 as the treatment was completed in a single sitting.

Two patients on Thermex 11 and one on Prostathermer developed mild urinary tract infection. No other significant complication was experienced with any of the machines.

The double-blind placebo-controlled trial

In the placebo-controlled trial patients were investigated and symptoms were scored as in the pilot study. Patients with chronic bacterial prostatitis were excluded from the study. Those with chronic abacterial prostatitis and prostatodynia were randomized into the placebo and the active treatment groups. The active group was treated with the Primus transrectal microwave hyperthermia machine in four sessions of 1 hour duration each spread over 2–3 weeks. The temperatures were raised to 43.8°C with a maximum power input of 40 W. The patients in the placebo group underwent a similar treatment protocol; however, though the transrectal probe was inserted the power setting was at 1 W and the maximum temperature was 37°C only. Postoperative assessment was done by one of the authors who was unaware of the treatment given. Since the patients were counselled before the treatment that they might not be able to appreciate any temperature changes, the placebo patients were not expecting any obvious heat effects. Direct questioning of the patients after the treatment confirmed the blind to be fairly well maintained in all the patients.

Results of the placebo trial

In this trial a similar assessment criteria to the pilot study has been adopted. The results are shown in Tables 8.5 and 8.6.

- Twenty-six patients have so far completed this trial. Thirteen patients were in the active group and 13 in the placebo group.
- Assessment at the end of treatment shows 9 out of the 13 patients in the active group (70%) showed greater than 50% improvement in their symptoms.
- In the placebo group 12 out of 13 patients (92%) showed no improvement, while one patient showed an improvement of more than 50% (placebo effect).
- In the active group 8 patients (62%) continued their improvement at 12 weeks. In the placebo group after the same period 11 patients (85%) were still without any change in their symptoms; however,

Table 8.5. Results of microwave hyperthermia versus placebo

	Improvement in treatment group ($n = 13$)		Improvement in placebo group ($n = 13$)	
Follow-up time	$<50\%$ No. (%)	$>50\%$ No. (%)	$<50\%$ No. (%)	$>50\%$ No. (%)
Immediate	4 (30)	9 (70)	12 (92)	1 (8)
6 weeks	4 (30)	9 (70)	12 (92)	1 (8)
12 weeks	5 (38)	8 (62)	11 (85)	2 (15)

Table 8.6. Microwave hyperthermia treatment versus placebo. Breakdown of the results, showing symptoms score improvement ($n = 13$)

	Treatment group				Placebo group			
Follow-up time	None No. (%)	25–50% No. (%)	51–75% No. (%)	76–100% No. (%)	None No. (%)	25–50% No. (%)	51–75% No. (%)	76–100% No. (%)
Immediate	2 (15)	2 (15)	8 (62.5)	1 (7.5)	11 (85)	1 (7.5)	1 (7.5)	0
6 weeks	2 (15)	2 (15)	8 (62.5)	1 (7.5)	11 (85)	1 (7.5)	1 (7.5)	0
12 weeks	4 (31)	1 (7.5)	7 (54)	1 (7.5)	11 (85)	0	1 (7.5)	1 (7.5)

2 patients (15%) showed greater than 50% improvement (placebo effect) at this stage.

- The early results of the placebo-controlled trial confirm the efficacy of this form of treatment, however, there is a placebo effect of about 15%.

Discussion

Assimilating the facts about the treatment of chronic prostatitis or 'prostatitis syndrome' it becomes apparent that the first essential is to correctly diagnose and then classify the condition into one of the three groups. Only then can a logical treatment policy be achieved. Chronic bacterial prostatitis should be treated with appropriate antibiotics, preferably one of the newer quinolones, which should then be continued for at least a period of 6 weeks. Chronic abacterial prostatitis and prostatodynia, however, require a different approach. Antibiotics in such patients are illogical and provide no significant benefit. Treatments should be directed in them at relaxing the external sphincteric musculature and the smooth muscles of the bladder neck and prostatic capsule. This can be achieved by alpha-adrenergic blockade or, as our work shows, more significant and lasting relief can be obtained by deep localized microwave hyperthermia. Stress is an important factor in some of these patients, and should be comprehensively investigated. Properly instituted stress therapy may provide useful alleviation of symptoms in such individuals. Symptomatic relief with non-steroidal anti-inflammatory drugs may be required and is a helpful adjuvant. The mode of action of microwave hyperthermia on the prostate is unclear. Perhaps there is a direct effect on the motor and sensory neural control to the prostate and the sphincteric mechanism. A normalization of the disturbed flow pattern along with relief of pain has been reported by Barnes *et al.* (1991a,b). This has been attributed to an effect on its complex neural control or on the sphincteric musculature.

Whatever the mode of action it is a useful treatment in a difficult condition. It is also useful to repeat the treatment should a relapse occur after an initial response.

It also becomes apparent from the results that patient selection, to exclude chronic bacterial prostatitis, will improve the outcome of the treatment. Moreover, although the relapse continues with time the beneficial effects of the treatment can be maintained for up to 2 years.

The early results of the placebo-controlled double-blind trial confirm the effectiveness of microwave hyperthermia in the treatment of chronic abacterial prostatitis and prostatodynia. As expected there is a placebo effect but the active treatment group shows a very significant improvement in the symptoms.

References

Aagaard J. & Madsen P.O. (1991) Bacterial prostatitis: new methods of treatment. *Urology*, **37** (Suppl. 3), 4–8.

Baert L., Mattelaer J. & Nollin de P. (1983) Treatment of chronic bacterial prostatitis by local injection of antibiotics into the prostate. *Urology*, **11**, 370–5.

Ball P. (1989) Long term use of quinolones and their safety. *Rev. Infect. Dis.*, **11**, 5, S1365–70.

Barnes D.G., Perlmutter A.P. & Watson G.M. (1991a) Transrectal hyperthermia in the benign painful prostate. *World J. Urol.*, **9**, 12–15.

Barnes D.G., Shah T.K., Perlmutter A.P. & Watson G.M. (1991b) Hyperthermia in the painful prostate. BAUS Annual Meeting, 28 June, Glasgow.

Barbalias G.A. (1990) Prostatodynia or painful male urethral syndrome? *Urology*, **36**, 146–53.

Barbalias G.A., Meares E.M. Jr. & Sant G.R. (1983) Prostatodynia: clinical and urodynamic characteristics. *J. Urol.*, **130**, 514–20.

Berger R.E., Krieger J.N., Kessler D., Ireton R.C., Close C., Holmes K.K. & Roberts P.L. (1989) Case control study of men with suspected chronic idiopathic prostatitis. *J. Urol.*, **141**, 328–31.

Buck A.C., Rees R.W. & Ebeling L. (1989) Treatment of chronic prostatitis and prostatodynia with pollen extract. *Br. J. Urol.*, **64**, 496–9.

Cheng H.J. & Huang G.G. (1987) Two balloon and four channel silicone rubber catheter for drug administration in the treatment of chronic bacterial prostatitis. *Eur. Urol.*, **13**, 116–7.

Doble A. & Carter S.S. (1989) Ultrasonographic findings in prostatitis. *Urol. Clin. North. Amer.*, **16**, 763–72.

Eykyn S., Bultitude M.I. & Lloyd Davies R.W. (1974) Prostatic calculi as a source of recurrent bacteriuria in the male. *Br. J. Urol.*, **46**, 527–35.

Fair W.R., Couch J. & Wehner N. (1976) Prostatic antibacterial factor. Identity and significance. *Urology*, **7**, 169–77.

Hellstorm W.J., Schmidt R.A., Lue T.F. & Tanagho E.A. (1987) Neuromuscular dysfunction in non-bacterial prostatitis. *Urology*, **30**, 183–8.

Ikeuchi T. (1990) Clinical studies on chronic prostatitis and prostatitis like syndrome. *Hinyokika Kiyo*, **36**, 561–8.

Jimenez-Cruz J.F., Tormo F.B. & Gomez J.G. (1988) Treatment of chronic prostatitis: intraprostatic antibiotic injections under echography control. *J. Urol.*, **139**, 967–70.

Krieger J.N. & Egan K.J. (1991) Comprehensive evaluation and treatment of 75 men referred to chronic prostatitis clinic. *Urology*, **38**, 11–19.

Kumamoto Y., Tsukamoto T., Sakai S., Guoro T., Maekwa S., Oguma K., Henmi I. *et al.* (1987) The therapeutic effect of norfloxacin on chronic prostatitis. *Hinyokika Kiyo*, **33**, 471–84.

Mackenzie A.R. (1986) Estrogen treatment of chronic abacterial prostatitis (letters). *Urology*, **27**, 574–5.

McNeal J.E. (1972) The prostate and prostatic urethra: A morphologic synthesis. *J. Urol.*, **107**, 1008–16.

Meares E.M. Jr. & Stamey T.A. (1968) Bacterialogic localization patterns in bacterial prostatitis and urethritis. *Invest. Urol.*, **5**, 492–518.

Meares E.M. Jr. (1973) Observations on the activity of trimethoprim–sulphamethoxazole in the prostate. *J. Infect. Dis.* (Suppl.) **128**, 679–85.

Meares E.M. Jr. (1974) Infection stones of the prostate gland: Laboratory diagnosis and clinical management. *Urology*, **4**, 560–70.

Meares E.M. Jr. (1975) Long term therapy of chronic bacterial prostatitis with trimethoprim–sulphamethoxazole. *Can. Med. Assoc. J.*, **112**, 22S–25S.

Meares E.M. Jr. (1980) Prostatitis syndromes: New perspectives old woes. *J. Urol.*, **123**, 141–7.

Meares E.M. Jr. (1987) Acute and chronic prostatitis: diagnosis and treatment. *Infect. Dis. Clin. North Amer.*, **1**, 855–73.

Meares G.M. Jr. & Barbalias G.A. (1983) Prostatitis: Bacterial, non-bacterial and prostatodynia. *Semin. Urol.*, **1**, 146–54.

Miller H.C. (1988) Stress prostatitis. *Urology*, **32**, 507–10.

Morikawa M., Tokunaka S., Yachuki S., Yamauchi K., Wakabayashi A. & Inagaki (1990) The therapeutic effect of norfloxacin on chronic prostatitis. *Hinyokika Kiyo*, **36**, 1253–7.

Nelson O.A. (1952) Impropriety of excessive prostatic massage. *Postgrad. Med.*, **12**, 82–4.

Ogawa A., Shimazaki J., Mitsuya H. *et al.* (1989) Clinical effects of terodiline hydrochloride on urinary frequency and sense of residual urine: a double blind clinical trial using flavoxate hydrochloride as a control. *Hinyokika Kiyo*, **34**, 739–53.

Orland S.M., Hanno P.M. & Wein A.J. (1985) Prostatitis, prostatosis and prostatodynia. *Urology*, **25**, 439–59.

Osborn D.E., George N.J., Rao P.N., Barnard R.J., Reading C., Marklow C. & Blacklock N.J. (1981) Prostatodynia physiological characteristics and rational management with muscle relaxants. *Br. J. Urol.*, **53**, 621–3.

Paulson D.F. & White R.D. (1978) Trimethoprim–sulphamethoxazole and minocycline HCl in the treatment of culture proved bacterial prostatitis. *J. Urol.*, **120**, 184–8.

Paulson D.F., Zinner N.R., Resnick M.I., Childs S.J., Love T. & Madsen P.O. (1986) Treatment of bacterial prostatitis. Comparison of cephalexin and minocycline. *Urology*, **27**, 379–87.

Remy G. (1990) Prostatitis. *Rev. Prat.*, **40**, 1285–8.

Segura J.W., Opitz J.L. & Greene L.F. (1979) Prostatosis, prostatitis or pelvic floor myalgia? *J. Urol.*, **122**, 168–9.

Servadio C., Leib Z. & Lev A. (1986) Further observations on the use of local hyperthermia for the treatment of prostate in man. *Eur. Urol.*, **12**, 38–40.

Servadio C., Leib Z. & Lev A. (1987) Diseases of prostate treated by local microwave hyperthermia. *Urology*, **30**, 97–9.

Shafik A. (1991) Anal submucosal injection: A new route for drug administration in chronic prostatitis: a new modality of treatment with report of eleven cases. *Urology*, **37**, 61–4.

Sinaki M., Merritt J.L. & Stillwell G.K. (1977) Tension myalgia of pelvic floor. *Mayo Clin. Proc.*, **52**, 717–21.

Siroki M.B., Goldstein I. & Krane R.J. (1981) Functional voiding disorders in men. *J. Urol.*, **126**, 200–4.

Smart C.J. & Jenkins J.D. (1973) The role of TURP in chronic prostatitis. *Br. J. Urol.*, **45**, 654–62.

Smart C.J., Jenkins J.D. & Llyod R.J. (1976) The painful prostate. *Br. J. Urol.*, **47**, 861–9.

Stamey T.A., Meares E.M. Jr. & Winningham D.G. (1970) Chronic bacterial prostatitis and the diffusion of drugs into the prostatic fluid. *J. Urol.*, **103**, 187–94.

Szolnoki G. & Keri V. (1989) Observations in the course of follow up Sumetrolin treated patients. *Ther. Hung.*, **37**, 154–9.

Thin R.N. & Simmons P.D. (1983) Review of four regimens for treatment of chronic non-bacterial prostatitis. *Br. J. Urol.*, **55**, 519–21.

Wedren H. (1987) Effects of sodium pantosanpolysulphate on symptoms related to chronic non-bacterial prostatitis. A double blind randomized study. *Scand. J. Urol. Nephrol.*, **21**, 81–8.

Wedren H. (1989) On chronic prostatitis with special studies of staphylococcal epidermidis. *Scand. J. Urol. Nephrol.* (suppl.) **123**, 1–36.

Winningham D.G. & Stamey T.A. (1968) Diffusion of antibiotics from plasma into prostatic fluid. *Nature*, **219**, 139–43.

Yerushalmi A. (1988) Localized, non-invasive deep microwave hyperthermia for the treatment of prostatic tumours: The first five years. *Cancer Res.*, **107**, 141–6.

9 Urethral and prostatic stents

E.J. MILROY

Introduction

The problems associated with implanting foreign materials within the lumen of the urinary tract, particularly in the bladder or urethra are well recognized. Catheters, indwelling stents or any material left in contact with urine will inevitably become infected and will encrust with phosphatic deposits from the urine. Although attempts have been made in the past to avoid these problems by using materials which either repel urine or are themselves inert, they have all failed to prevent them completely. It has also been found that once infection and incrustation have occurred they are impossible to eradicate without removing the implanted material.

These problems, together with the difficulty of preventing movement of implanted material in the lower urinary tract (either causing the implant to be expelled from the urethra or causing it to encroach on the sphincter mechanisms and cause incontinence), have relegated implanted lower urinary tract devices to the temporary relief of obstruction while awaiting more definitive treatment.

A major breakthrough was made when it was found that woven mesh stent devices manufactured of fine corrosion-resistant 'superalloy' wire would cover with normal urothelium after implantation within the urethra, excluding the foreign material from contact with urine and thereby avoiding complications of infection and incrustation (Milroy *et al.*, 1988; Sarramon *et al.*, 1989).

Prostatic stents

Temporary

The first description of an indwelling urethral device to replace a permanent urethral catheter in the treatment of prostate obstruction was a report by Fabian (1980) of what he called a 'partial catheter' or 'urological spiral'. This device consists of a closely coiled spiral of stainless steel wire tapered at the inner end to allow for its insertion into the urethra. At the outer end of the coil a single strand of wire passes through the sphincter with another smaller coil lying outside the distal sphincter mechanism allowing for adjustment in position and removal of the stent. Problems were experienced with difficulty in insertion, movement of the stent and incrustation, although in general it worked well as a temporary device. This stent is now marketed by Porges as the 'Urospiral'.

A Danish company (Engineers and Doctors) have since developed a modification of the Fabian spiral. This device consists of the same close-coiled spiral of wire but this is now gold-plated to reduce the amount of incrustation (Fig. 9.1). Introduction of the device is made easier by a detachable catheter which allows the stent to be passed under local anaesthetic under transrectal ultrasound control. Good results have been obtained with the use of this device, particularly in patients with acute urinary retention unfit for surgery (Nordling *et al.*, 1989). There are still occasional problems with the insertion of the device and although problems of infection and incrustation are reduced they will inevitably still occur, unless the device is regularly changed, because the device remains in constant contact with urine. Harrison & De Souza (1990) reported their experience in 30 unfit patients, most with urinary retention, with successful relief of obstruction in 80% of patients with acute retention. Although the device is made in a variety of sizes the diameter of each device is fixed and it has no intrinsic means of fixing itself within the prostatic urethra. This undoubtedly accounts for a number of cases of the stent moving position either into the bladder or distally to cause incontinence. A report of the urodynamic evaluation of eight patients with this device was made by Nielsen *et al.* (1989). They found that the stent allowed unobstructed voiding in the majority of their patients. There are always going to be problems in the patients with chronic retention

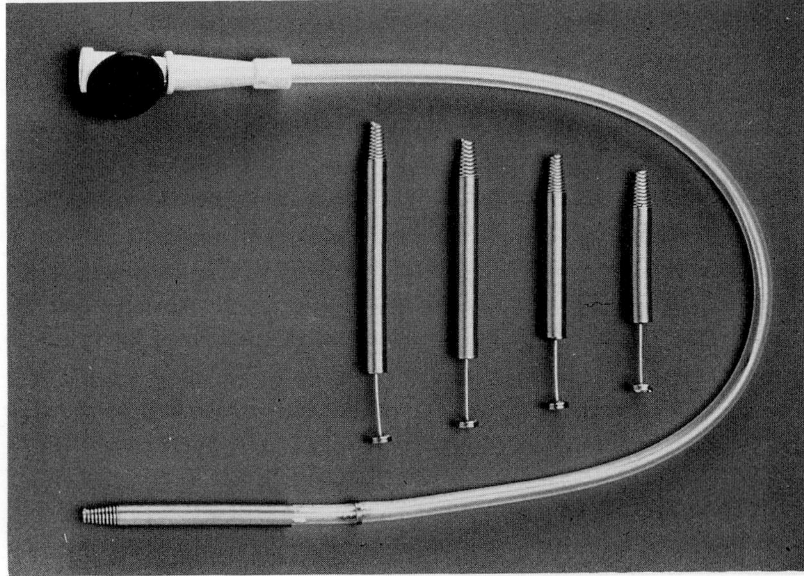

Fig. 9.1. The Prostakath[R] urethral stent.

and severely reduced detrusor function and as with any intra-urethral device a number of patients will continue to suffer irritative symptoms of frequency and urgency while the device is in place.

Nissenkorn described a short double Malecot (16 French) polyurethane catheter which he described introducing into the prostatic urethra in patients with acute urinary retention (Nissenkorn, 1989; Nissenkorn & Richter, 1990). The catheter is made in three lengths, 45, 55, and 60 mm, and is introduced into the prostatic urethra under local anaesthetic through a cystoscope sheath, the length of the prostatic urethra having been measured endoscopically or by ultrasound (Fig. 9.2). The inner Malecot end of the device lies within the bladder at the bladder neck and the distal end should lie just distal to the verumontanum. A nylon suture is threaded through the distal end of the device and emerges from the urethra. This can be used to remove the device if unsatisfactory. If the device is to be left in place the nylon can be cut short and left lying in the anterior urethra. All 14 patients were able to void after insertion of the catheter and were continent. A number suffered from frequency or urgency and three devices had to be removed. This device is only intended for temporary use, although it has been left in place for up to 18 weeks without complication.

Permanent stents

We first used the Urolume* Wallstent[R] nearly 4 years ago for the treatment of recurrent bulbar urethral stricture. This proved so successful that we decided to test its effectiveness in the prostatic urethra

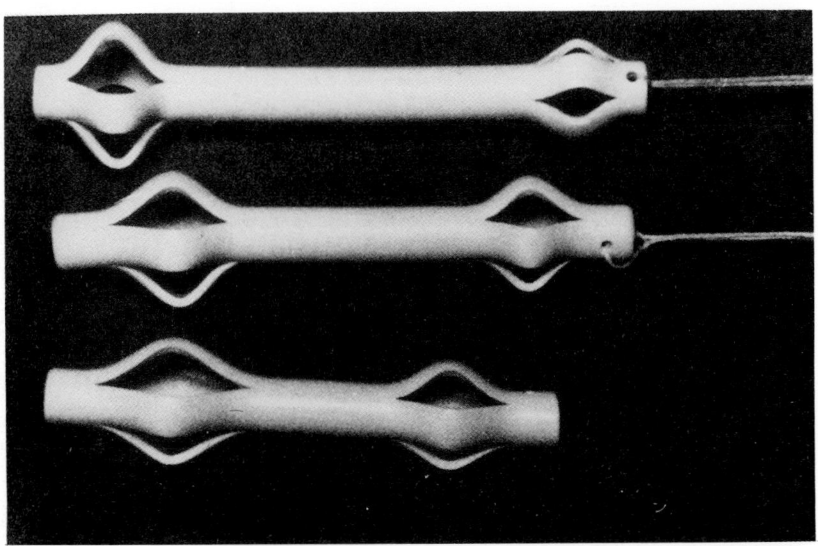

Fig. 9.2. Nissenkorn catheter.

* Urethral and prostate Wallstents[R] are now manufactured and marketed as the 'Urolume[R]' by American Medical Systems, Minnesota, USA.

for the relief of acute retention and severe urinary symptoms from prostate obstruction (Chapple *et al.*, 1990).

The Wallstent^{R} is a woven tubular mesh of corrosion-resistant 'superalloy' wire and is manufactured in various lengths and diameters (Fig. 9.3); when it is expanded from its delivery system the stent is stable though flexible. The stent, originally invented by Hans Wallsten of Medinvent*, Lausanne, Switzerland, was first designed for endovascular use where it has been successfully employed for nearly 6 years in the prevention of restenosis after transluminal angioplasty (Sigwart *et al.*, 1987).

The original system we used in the urinary tract was modified from that developed for endovascular use and consists of a small-diameter (9 F) delivery catheter (Fig. 9.4). A doubled-over plastic membrane holds the stent in a compressed and elongated form. The double membrane system is then pressurized to 3 atmospheres (303 kPa), after which the outer layer of membrane can be progressively withdrawn to allow the stent to expand when it has been positioned within the previously dilated urethral stricture or prostate. The expansile force of the mesh then holds it in position, preventing any possibility of displacement of the stent and, because of the fine wire structure of the mesh, allowing urothelium to grow over the implanted material whilst holding open the urethra.

We have recently developed, with Hans Wallsten, a new delivery system for the stent which consists of an endoscopic device produced

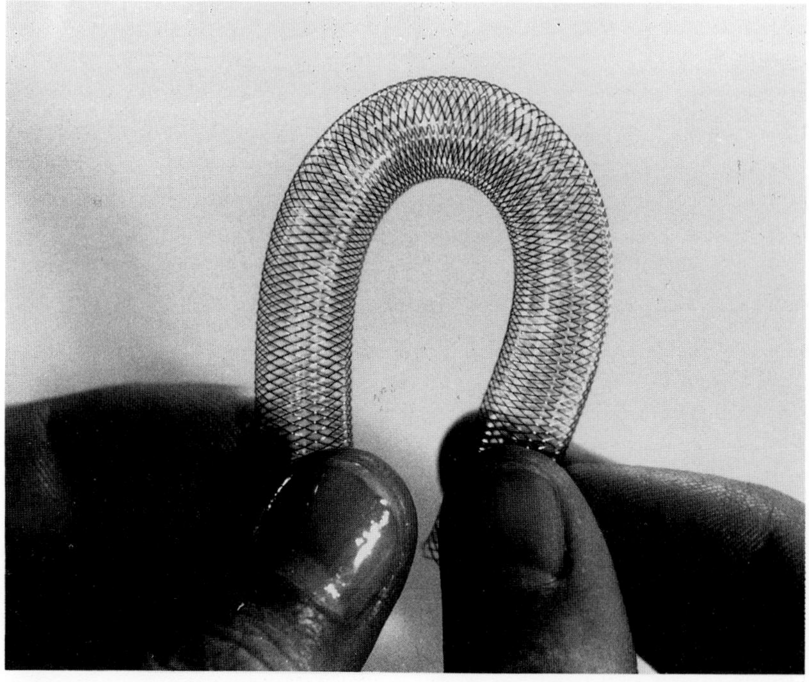

Fig. 9.3. American Medical Systems Urolume^{R} urethral Wallstent^{R}.

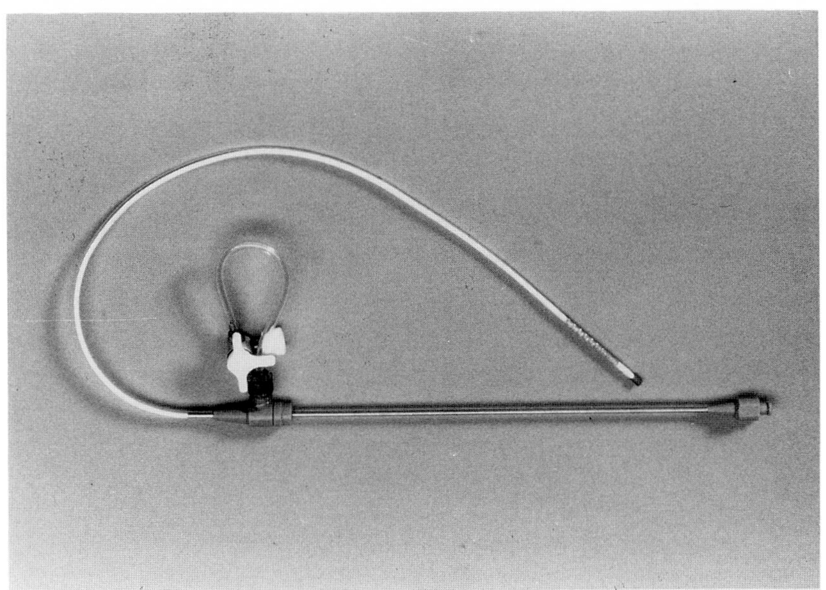

Fig. 9.4. Original delivery system for Wallstent[R].

specifically for the urologist (Fig. 9.5). Using this new device, the difficulties of the stent shortening as it expands from its small-diameter delivery catheter are considerably reduced. A standard 0° telescope is inserted down the centre of the device and may be moved longitudinally, enabling the full extent of the stent to be observed as it opens, ensuring that both ends of the stent are positioned correctly (Fig. 9.6). The device includes a locking mechanism preventing final deployment of the stent until correct positioning has been achieved. Until this lock is released the stent can be recovered into the delivery system by advancing the outer sheath over the stent. This allows repositioning before the stent is reopened and finally deployed. The outer sheath of this new delivery system measures 21 F.

Another great advantage of this permanent stent is that the internal diameter of the stent is large enough to permit endoscopic surgery if necessary. Most of the stents we have used for urethral strictures and prostate obstruction have been 14 mm diameter (43 F) in lengths of 20 or 30 mm. These dimensions are measured with the stent unconstrained and exerting no radial force. It must be emphasized that when used in the urethra the diameter is smaller than this, exerting a radial force against the urethra; the length of the stent in this situation is correspondingly greater.

Experimental work

First experimental work using this stent in the blood vessels of experimental animals was carried out by Professor J.P. Sarramon (pers.

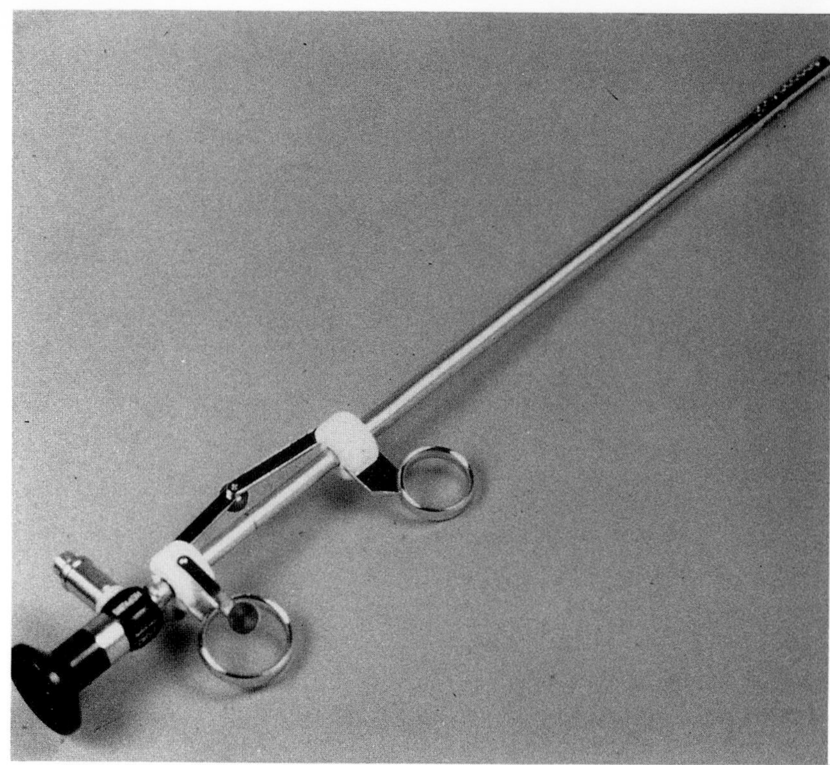

Fig. 9.5. New introducer for Wallstent[R].

comm.) and he demonstrated rapid covering of the stent with normal endothelium. In collaboration with Professor Sarramon, Toulouse, France, we then decided to use the stent in the lower urinary tract and implanted the Wallstent[R] into the normal posterior urethra of a number of male dogs. Urethral stents 4.5 mm diameter, 10 mm length were inserted into the dogs' urethras using the standard original small-diameter delivery catheter. The stents were positioned to lie in the bulbar part of the urethra just proximal to the os penis. Urethras from the dogs were examined between 2 and 12 months after implantation. Scanning electron microscopy showed virtually complete covering of the stent between 6 and 12 months after insertion. Histological examination of deeper tissues showed remarkably little inflammation or fibrosis (Milroy *et al.*, 1988; Sarramon *et al.*, 1989).

Clinical experience

Urethral strictures

We have now treated over 60 patients with urethral strictures during the last 3 years and the stent has been remarkably successful although the follow-up is still rather short. All bulbar strictures had failed at

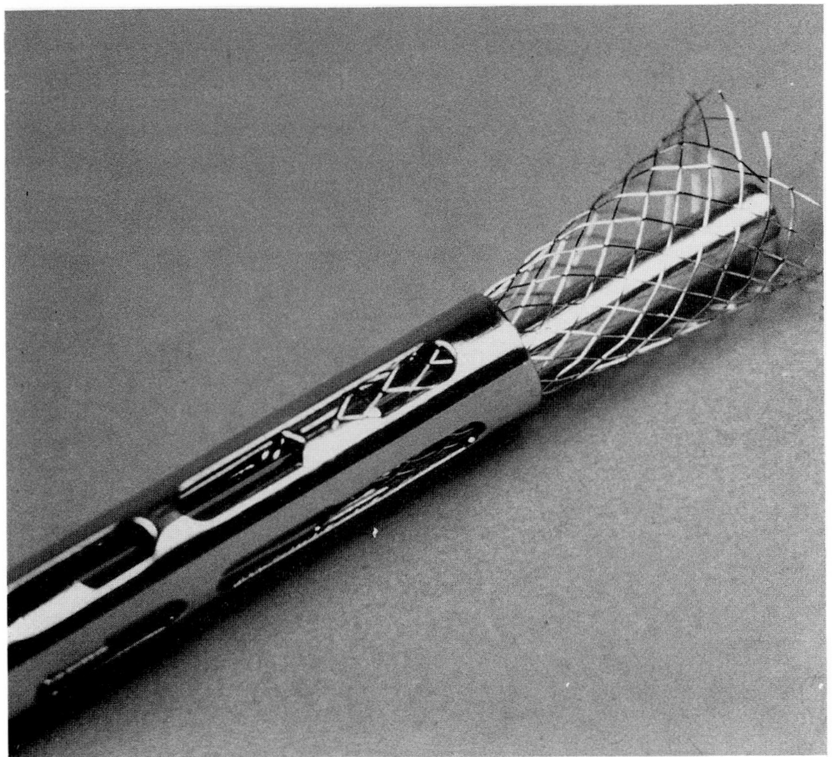

Fig. 9.6. Close-up view of stent within sheath of introducer. Note telescope within lumen of stent.

least two endoscopic urethrotomies; in addition eight of them had recurred after urethroplasty procedures. The stents have all epithelialized within 4–6 months of implantation although this takes longer in patients after urethroplasty surgery. The stents stimulate a considerable hyperplastic reaction in a few patients, but the only occasions we have seen obstruction within the lumen of the stent have been in patients with complete traumatic rupture strictures and, very occasionally, from a particularly florid hyperplastic reaction after failed urethroplasty; the hyperplastic reaction will usually settle within 1 year. Eight patients have had a recurrence of part of the original stricture when the stent was misplaced at the original insertion. In all cases this has been treated successfully with an additional overlapping stent. Complications have been few. We have had no problems with movement of the stent or incrustation, and only one stent has become infected, but this settled without difficulty following a standard course of antibiotics. Discomfort from the stent is temporary and the only other problem patients have experienced is the occasional passage of a few drops of urine with coughing and straining presumably from the release of a small amount of urine contained within the lumen of the stent.

We have had some experience of treating membranous urethral

strictures. As mentioned already complete urethral rupture in this area can lead to obstruction within the lumen of the stent and this device is not recommended at this stage for treating traumatic strictures. Other membranous urethral strictures can be treated with the subsequent implantation of an artificial urinary sphincter if the bladder neck is incompetent.

There is no doubt that the Wallstent[R] is an excellent treatment for many difficult recurrent urethral strictures, particularly those lying within the bulbar membranous urethra. Longer follow-up is necessary before it will be possible to be definitive about the final place of this treatment in the primary management of urethral strictures, but this device should certainly be considered as an effective alternative if other procedures have failed (Milroy *et al.*, 1989a,b).

Other indications

In conjunction with Julian Shah we have had considerable experience of using this device in patients with traumatic high cervical spinal injuries causing tetraplegia and dyssynergic sphincters. These patients have all had high-pressure voiding and were unsuitable for intermittent catheterization. Stents were inserted using the same device as that used for urethral strictures, and the procedure was notable for its simplicity and lack of complications. All patients were fully assessed urodynamically before and after the procedure and all were voiding with lower detrusor pressures, and, if not voiding to completion, were leaving smaller residual urines. It is notable that this group of patients were far more enthusiastic about the original stent and its subsequent result than they were about endoscopic sphincterotomy, four of them having undergone previous unsuccessful sphincterotomy procedures (Shaw *et al.*, 1990).

The stent has also been used successfully for the treatment of biliary strictures (Dick *et al.*, 1989) and in a number of cases of tracheal and oesophageal obstruction. The hyperplastic reaction seen when the stent is first inserted has prevented widespread use of the device in ureteric obstruction, although early clinical results have been promising.

Prostate obstruction

We have developed two techniques for inserting the Wallstent[R] into the prostatic urethra. As these techniques were developed for use in unfit patients all prostate stents have been inserted using local urethral lignocaine with additional intravenous short-acting benzodiazepine as necessary. With a few of the more anxious patients we have used a spinal anaesthetic. The original technique for the prostate Wallstent[R] used transrectal ultrasound guidance. After we had developed the new endoscopic delivery system for the stent we inserted prostate stents under direct endoscopic control, again using local anaesthetic but without the need for X-ray or ultrasound assistance.

Ultrasound-guided technique

We used the ultrasound-guided technique for the first 24 prostate stents inserted. The patient lies in the left lateral position on an X-ray table and after local urethral anaesthetic has been administered a careful cystourethroscopy is carried out using a flexible cystoscope. The transrectal ultrasound probe is then inserted and the position of the bladder neck, verumontanum and distal sphincter mechanism are identified with the ultrasound probe and confirmed using a flexible cystoscope. The length of the prostatic urethra is then measured using ultrasound and the correct length of Wallstent^{R} on its small-diameter delivery system (see Fig. 9.4) is selected. A guide wire is passed down the instrument channel of the flexible cystoscope into the bladder and the cystoscope removed. After checking the mechanism and function of the double membrane system holding the compressed and elongated stent in position the delivery system catheter is threaded over the guide wire into the bladder. The double membrane system is then pressurized through the side arm with normal saline to 3 atmospheres (303 kPa) and the first third of the stent is then opened by pulling back the outer part of the delivery system mechanism, withdrawing the outer layer of the compressing membrane from the stent. The delivery catheter is then slowly pulled back until the partially opened stent can be seen on the ultrasound screen (Fig. 9.7). The membranes are now depressurized to prevent further opening of the stent whilst the catheter system is slowly withdrawn so that the inner open end of the stent can be positioned to lie just at the bladder neck using ultrasound guidance. When correctly positioned the membrane system is pressurized once more and the stent fully deployed by peeling back the membrane completely. Providing the stent has expanded fully and is in a satisfactory position the delivery catheter and guide wire are removed. The final position of the stent can then be checked using the flexible cystoscope. The patient is allowed to empty his bladder normally and no urethral catheter is left in position. Patients with chronic retention and others in whom a suprapubic catheter had been inserted to relieve acute retention have the suprapubic catheter left in position in order to monitor residual urine following stent insertion.

In 12 patients the stent failed to expand fully on deployment using this original delivery system and in these a 12 mm diameter dilating balloon catheter was passed over the guide wire and inflated within the lumen of the stent. We have had no problems with stents moving within the prostatic urethra once they have been deployed. The self-expanding properties of the wire mesh hold it firmly against the wall of the urethra.

The major problem with this ultrasound-guided system is in the final positioning of the stent. Once the membrane system has started withdrawing allowing the stent to open, it cannot be pushed back to compress the stent once more. In three patients the whole system had to be removed from the urethra because of inaccurate initial positioning of the stent too far distally down the prostatic urethra. This is easily accomplished by passing an open-ended plastic neoplex catheter over the whole stent-carrying mechanism after cutting off the outer pressurizing and deploying mechanism. The neoplex catheter is then advanced over the partially open stent, compressing it and allowing the stent delivery system and the neoplex catheter to be removed from the urethra together. This, of course, destroys the mechanism of the delivery system and another stent and delivery catheter need to be used for the patient. The other problem with this delivery system in the prostate is that once the final position at the bladder neck has been determined it is impossible to be absolutely sure where the distal end of the stent will lie. Of course, if the ultrasound measurements have been made correctly and the stent expands fully there will be no problem, but if the stent fails to open completely the distal end of the stent may lie within the sphincter area of the urethra. It is in this situation that balloon dilatation has proved useful in order to expand the stent fully. In one patient inaccurate prostate measurements were taken, causing too large a stent to be implanted. The stent opened fully, but was lying within the membranous urethra causing incontinence. The stent was later removed without difficulty and normal continence was regained.

In spite of the problems with the ultrasound guidance system it remains a useful technique for patients whose immobility or other medical conditions prevent them getting into the lithotomy position which is necessary for the endoscopic delivery technique.

Endoscopic technique

Because of difficulties experienced with the ultrasound-guided technique we have used the new endoscopic delivery system (Fig. 9.5) for the last 21 prostate stents we have inserted. Using this technique more accurate positioning of the stent can be assured.

Urethral anaesthesia and intravenous sedation are given and the patient placed in the extended lithotomy position. A cystoscopy is carried out to check for bladder pathology and the length of the prostatic urethra, from bladder neck to verumontanum, is measured using a calibrated ureteric catheter. Alternatively, the prostate length can be measured before stent insertion using transrectal ultrasound. A stent of an appropriate length is then selected on its endoscopic delivery system and is introduced into the prostatic urethra under direct vision using a standard Stortz 0° telescope. The first safety lock, which prevents premature opening of the stent as the device is passed down the urethra, is then removed and the stent is deployed within the prostatic urethra under direct vision by pulling back the outer sheath from the stent and allowing it to expand. Once the sheath has been pulled back to the second safety lock, the final position of the stent can be checked by moving the telescope along the length of the stent within the prostatic urethra. If the position of the stent is not correct, the outer sheath can be pushed back over the stent which will then close inside the sheath allowing repositioning as necessary. The inner end of the stent should lie just at the bladder neck, and at the outer end the distal margin of the lateral lobes and the verumontanum can be seen through the slots cut in the outer sheath of the delivery system. Once the final position is correct the safety lock is removed and the stent will spring open into its final position. The introducing sheath may then be removed and if necessary the stent can be examined endoscopically using a standard cystoscope. Great care must, however, be taken at this stage not to damage the wires of the distal part of the stent with the cystoscope.

Results

We have treated 45 patients with prostate obstruction using the urethral Wallstent[R]. Thirty-two patients presented with acute retention (Table 9.1). Thirty-nine prostates were benign. Forty-two patients are fully satisfied with the stent and are passing urine normally with significantly reduced residual urines. Wherever possible urodynamic videocystograms have been carried out before stent insertion and 3–6 months post-operatively. Post-operative studies have not been possible on a number of these patients because of increasingly severe medical problems which prevented prostate surgery when they first presented. The American Society of Anesthesiology's grading of these patients is shown in Table 9.2.

All patients suffered frequency urgency and occasional urge incontinence following stent insertion but this settled in all but two patients, both of whom have persistent severe detrusor instability. Six patients failed to pass urine immediately after stent insertion, necessitating

Table 9.1. Patients with prostate obstruction using urethral Wallstent[R]

45 patients
32 acute retention
7 chronic retention
3 severe symptoms
3 symptoms prostate/Parkinson's disease symptoms (therapeutic trial)
39 benign
6 malignant
Mean age 74.8 (range 49–95 years)

Table 9.2. Prostate stents: patient fitness status*

1 healthy	2 patients
2 mild systemic disease	5 patients
3 severe disease	15 patients
4 threat to life	23 patients
5 moribund	0 patients

* American Society of Anesthesiology's grading system

suprapubic catheterization. Voiding commenced in all these without difficulty during the next 2 to 3 days, and all suprapubic catheters (except one inserted pre-operatively for chronic retention and advanced prostate cancer) were removed by 6 weeks. Stents seem to cause remarkably few other symptoms and no patient has experienced pain unless associated with a urinary infection. Three of our patients experienced urinary infections after insertion of the stent but these all settled with a standard course of antibiotics and did not affect healing of the stent (Fig. 9.7).

In addition to urodynamic evaluation, wherever possible we have carried out regular cystoscopy under local anaesthetic to check on

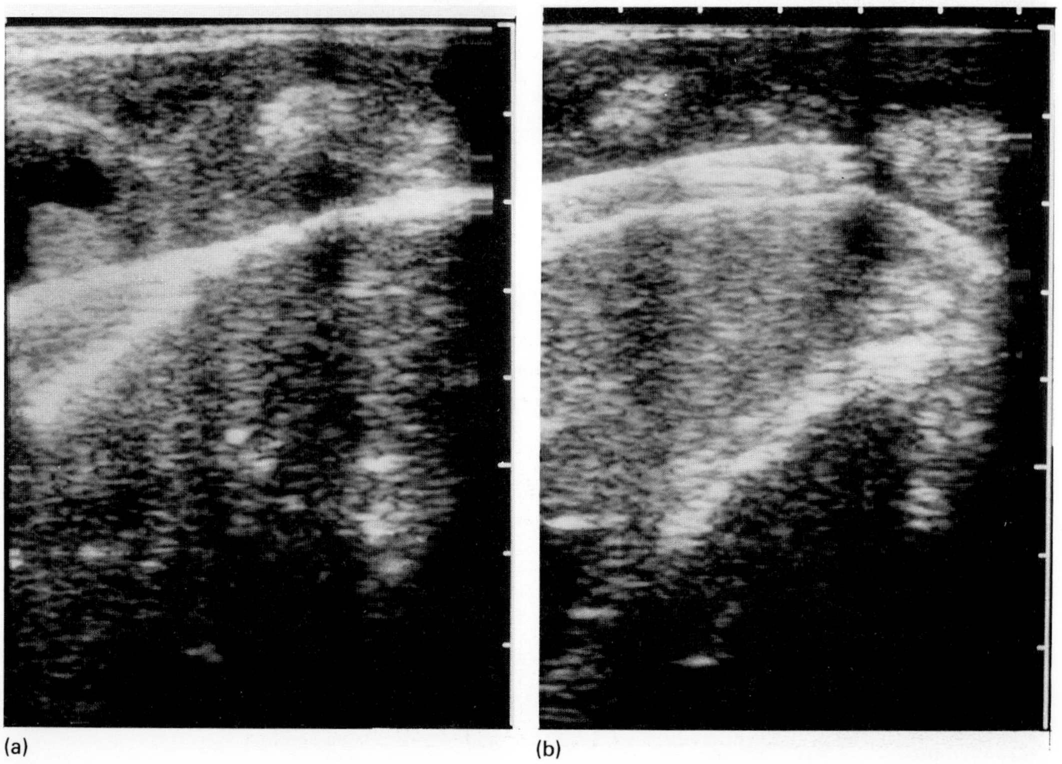

Fig. 9.7. (a) Transrectal ultrasound showing partially open stent at bladder neck. (b) Stent fully open within prostate.

healing of the stent. The stent seems to cover with urothelium in exactly the same way as the stents used for urethral strictures. There is a variable hyperplastic reaction (Fig. 9.8) which seems to last for longer in the prostate stents than in those used in the urethra, but does eventually seem to settle between 12 and 18 months after insertion (Fig. 9.9). We have seen no incrustation of the stents within the prostatic urethra. In a few of our earlier patients some small areas of the wire mesh were left lying within the bladder proximal to the bladder neck and in these patients fine incrustation of the wires can sometimes be seen after 6–12 months, although none of these stents have yet caused problems or needed removing.

As detailed above, three stents had to be removed before full deployment when we were using the rolling membrane catheter delivery system. All these patients had another stent inserted immediately without difficulty and with good results. Five other stents have been removed subsequent to deployment. Four of these were removed before full epithelialization. In these patients the stent can be removed without difficulty by grasping the stent at the bladder neck and pushing it into the bladder using standard grasping alligator

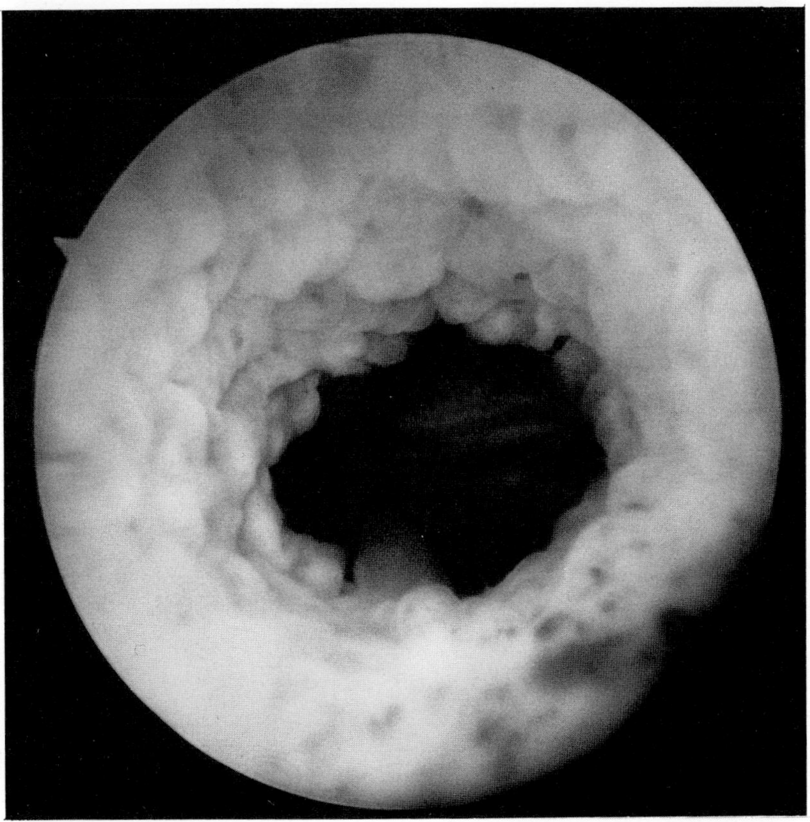

Fig. 9.8. Endoscopic appearance of prostate stent covered with hyperplastic urothelium 5 months after insertion. Patient has no symptoms.

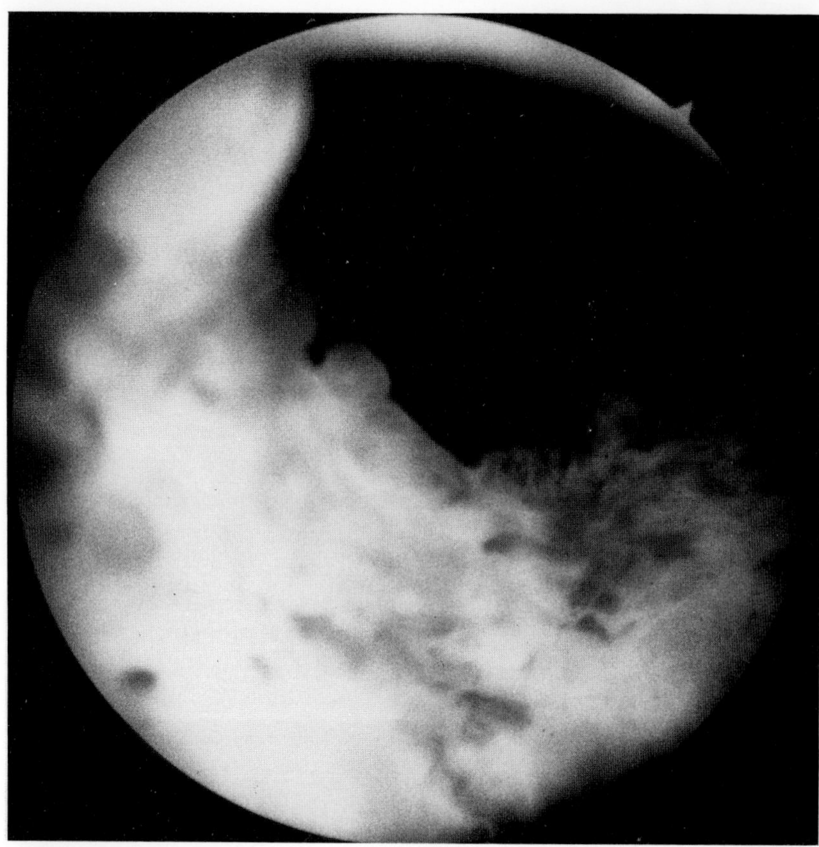

Fig. 9.9. Appearance of prostate stent 1 year after insertion. Stent covered, little hyperplasia remaining.

forceps. The stent can then be pulled into a large resectoscope sheath or simply pulled out through the urethra. As the stent is pulled it lengthens and narrows causing remarkably little damage to the distal urethra as it is pulled out. One stent was removed 11 months after implantation at the request of the patient because of persistence of severe detrusor instability. The somewhat hyperplastic lining epithelium was resected endoscopically without difficulty and the stent pushed into the bladder and removed as described above. The patient has needless to say not improved but he has, perhaps understandably, declined further treatment.

Several patients have noticed intermittent haematuria for the first 3–6 months and one of these presented with clot retention 3 months after implantation. This was treated with suprapubic catheterization and spontaneous voiding recommenced 48 hours later with cessation of the bleeding and no further symptoms.

No patient has reported any change in potency as a result of stent insertion, although it must be appreciated that the majority of these patients were elderly and suffering from severe chest and heart disease, preventing normal sexual intercourse. Most of those few patients having regular sexual intercourse report retrograde ejaculation, although it is interesting that two state that normal ejaculation has been maintained. The mean age of the patients is 74.8 years (range 49–95). The mean follow-up is 10.6 months (range 4–17).

Other permanent prostate stents

A number of other companies are in the process of trying to perfect endoscopically delivered prostate stents using endoscopic, ultrasound, or X-ray guidance. At the present time only one of these has reached the stage of early clinical trials. This stent is produced by Advanced Surgical Intervention Inc., San Clemente, California, and consists of a titanium mesh structure loaded on a prostate balloon dilatation system which can be deployed using either X-ray, ultrasound, or direct endoscopic control. The balloon is positioned within the prostatic urethra and as it expands the balloon forces open the titanium mesh into the prostatic urethra. Once the stent has expanded the balloon is deflated and removed. Unlike the Medinvent stent this stent has no intrinsic spring radial force, the diameter being fixed by the inflation of the 12 mm diameter balloon to approximately 32 F. The structure of the mesh is quite different from that of the Medinvent woven wire mesh structure. The ASI stent is an open framework of malleable titanium, the borders of the frame being larger in cross-sectional area than the fine wire of the Medinvent stent. This ASI stent (Fig. 9.10) certainly seems to work well in clinical trials in patients with acute retention, although it is too early to know how well it covers with epithelium and stabilizes.

Indications for prostate stents

Since the recent anxieties about the long-term results of prostate surgery (Roos *et al.*, 1989) there has been increasing interest both in the medical profession and more importantly amongst a well-informed general public in alternative treatments for prostate obstruction. It is particularly important that urologists with their knowledge, training and experience in treating diseases of the prostate gland should remain in the forefront of the development of new treatments.

There is no doubt that in the elderly and unfit patient for whom prostate surgery would be a major risk and for whom pharmacological treatment may cause unacceptable side-effects some form of prostate stenting to relieve acute retention or severe prostate symptoms offers an entirely justified and ideal alternative, providing the treatment can be carried out rapidly and uses local anaesthesia (Williams *et al.*, 1989; Chapple *et al.*, 1990). Included in this group may be patients who for one reason or another refuse prostate surgery and other forms of treatment. Until other new treatments are fully assessed and evaluated

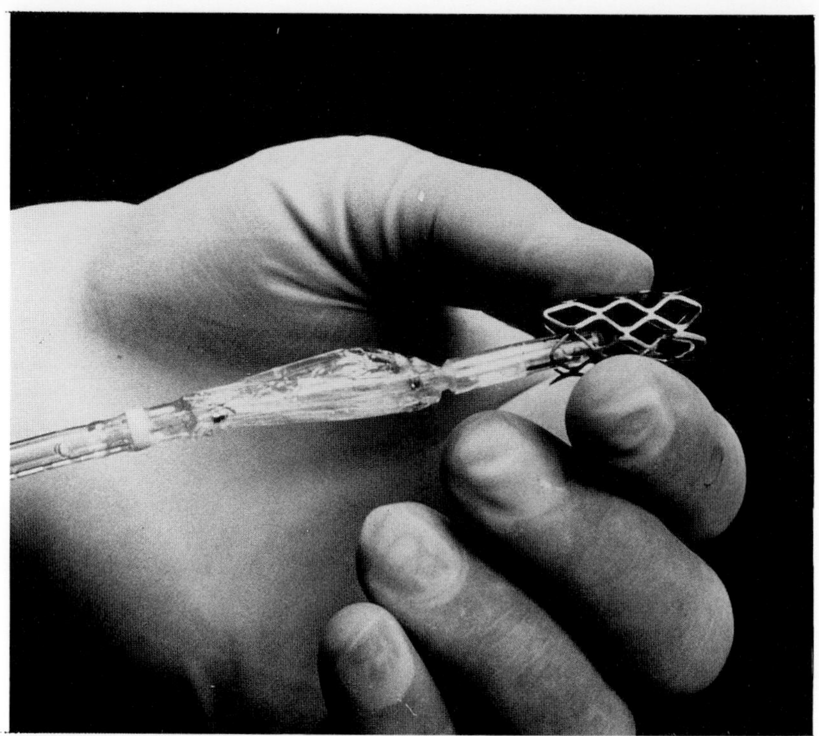

Fig. 9.10. ASI stent with balloon catheter.

there will remain in many parts of the world long waiting lists for prostate surgery. These patients are particularly suited to the various temporary prostate stents which are in general less expensive than the permanent stents.

Finally, we have used the Wallstent^R in what might be called a therapeutic trial in three patients with Parkinson's disease who have urinary symptoms which are difficult to distinguish symptomatically and urodynamically between those caused by the Parkinson's disease and possible prostate obstruction. Insertion of a prostate stent relieves any prostate obstruction. If the patient's symptoms and urodynamic results improve the stent can be left in position. If there is no improvement the stent can easily be removed. In our three patients the patient's symptoms improved as did their urodynamic results and the stents were left in place.

Future developments

There is no doubt that simple mechanical devices to hold open the obstructed prostatic urethra will continue to play an important part at least in the elderly unfit patient, and possibly in far larger groups of patients. Improvements can undoubtedly be made in delivery systems of the stents and possibly also in their structure, both to aid more accurate positioning within the prostatic urethra, and to encourage rapid and uncomplicated epithelial covering of the stent. This epithelial covering is vital to prevent incrustation and infection, which will always occur with any foreign body left in contact with urine.

The long-term stability of the permanent stents within the body cannot of course be determined at the present time because of the short time they have been in use. The alloy used in the Wallstent^R is tried and tested and is known to be well tolerated within the body. After a period of 20 years or so corrosion and fragmentation of the metal may tend to occur in body fluids. This is not likely to be a problem in patients with short life expectancy for whom this stent is ideal, but in any case any fragments would be totally encapsulated by surrounding tissues and any accumulation of corrosion products is unlikely to occur because of the thin covering of urothelium. The lines of force in the structure of the stent are such that any fragmentation of the wires would tend to move the fragments outwards rather than inwards and it is unlikely than any damage would occur from this. Although other metals and alloys may be less prone to fragmentation, corrosion will still occur to some extent within body fluids, but again is unlikely to be a serious problem.

Conclusion

Temporary prostate stents inserted under local anaesthesia offer an excellent alternative for short-term relief of acute retention or severe prostate symptoms in patients with a short life expectancy or awaiting prostate surgery. They cannot, however, be left in place for long periods of time without changing the stent. Permanently implanted prostate stents which cover with epithelium within the prostatic urethra offer the possibility of a permanent, simple, safe and effective alternative to prostate surgery.

References

Chapple C.R., Milroy E.J.G. & Rickards D. (1990) Permanently implanted urethral stents for prostate obstruction in the unfit patient. *Brit. J. Urol.*, **66**, 58–65.

Dick R., Gillams A., Dooley J.S. & Hobbs K.E.F. (1989) Stainless steel mesh stents for biliary strictures. *J. Intervent. Radiol.*, **4**, 95–8.

Fabian K.M. (1980) Der intraprostatische 'Partielle Katheter' (Urologische Spirale). *Urologe A*, **19**, 236–8.

Harrison N.W. & De Souza J.V. (1990) Prostate stenting for outflow obstruction. *Brit. J. Urol.*, **65**, 192–6.

Milroy E.J.G., Chapple C.R., Cooper J.E., Eldin A., Wallsten H., Seddon A.M. & Rowles P.M. (1988) A new treatment for urethral strictures. *Lancet*, **1**, 1424–7.

Milroy E.J.G., Chapple C.R., Eldin A. & Wallsten H. (1989a) A new stent for the treatment of urethral strictures. *Brit. J. Urol.*, **63**, 392–6.

Milroy E.J.G., Chapple C.R., Eldin A. & Wallsten H. (1989b) A new treatment for urethral strictures: a permanently implanted urethral stent. *J. Urol.*, **141**, 1120–2.

Nielsen K.K., Kromann-Andersen B. & Nording J. (1989) Relationship between detrusor pressure and urinary flow rate in males with an intra-urethral prostatic spiral. *Brit. J. Urol.*, **64**, 275–9.

Nissenkorn I. (1989) Experience with a new self retaining intraurethral catheter in patients with urinary retention. *J. Urol.*, **142**, 92–4.

Nissenkorn I. & Richter S. (1990) A self retaining intra-urethral device. *Brit. J. Urol.*, **65**, 197–200.

Nordling J., Holm H.H., Klarskov P., Nielson K.K. & Andersen J.T. (1989) Intraprostatic spiral: new device for insertion with patient under local anaesthetic and with ultrasonic guidance with three months of follow up. *J. Urol.*, **142**, 756–8.

Roos N.P., Wennberg J.E., Malenka D.J., Fisher E.S., McPherson K., Andersen T.F., Cohen M.M. & Romsey E. (1989) Mortality and reoperation after open and transurethral resection of the prostate for benign prostatic hyperplasia. *N. Engl. J. Med.*, **320**, 1120–4.

Sarramon J.P., Joffre F., Rischmann P., Rousseau H., Eldin A. & Wallstent H. (1989) Prosthese endourethrale wallstent dans les stenoses recidivantes de l'urethre. *Ann. Urol.*, **23**, 383–7.

Shaw P.J.R., Milroy E.J.G. & Eldin A. (1990) Permanent external sphincter stents in spinal injured patients. *Brit. J. Urol.*, **66**, 297–302.

Sigwart U., Puel J., Mirkovitch V., Joffre F. & Kappenberger L. (1987) Intravascular stents to prevent occlusion and restenosis after transluminal angioplasty. *N. Engl. J. Med.*, **316**, 701–6.

Williams G., Jager R., McLoughlin L., el Din A., Machan L., Gill K., Asopa R. & Adam A. (1989) Use of stents for treating obstruction of urinary outflow in patients unfit for surgery. *Brit. Med. J.*, **298**, 1429.

10 Transurethral resection of the prostate under sedation and local anaesthesia (sedoanalgesia)

B.R.P. BIRCH AND R.A. MILLER

Introduction

General

Transurethral resection of the prostate (TURP) constitutes the major part of the urologist's work load. Performed under general or regional anaesthesia, it provides good symptomatic relief for patients presenting with outflow obstruction (Graverson *et al.*, 1989). Both the mortality and morbidity of transurethral resection performed in this way are low although noted to increase with increasing age of the patient (Wyatt *et al.*, 1989).

There has been increasing interest directed towards techniques which are either non-invasive or minimally invasive and can be performed under local anaesthesia (topically or by infiltration). Currently available alternatives to conventional TURP include balloon dilatation (Gill *et al.*, 1989), closed commissurotomy (Shafik, 1988), microwave hypothermia (Lindner *et al.*, 1987; Servadio *et al.*, 1987), endoprostatic stents (Fabian, 1978; Milroy *et al.*, 1989), alpha-adrenergic blockade (Caine *et al.*, 1978; Ferrie & Paterson, 1987; Kirby *et al.*, 1987), phenol injection (Angell, 1969), cytotoxic agents (Wei & Zhou, 1987) and endocrine manipulation using LHRH (luteinizing-hormone-releasing hormone) agonists (Keane *et al.*, 1988), anti-androgens (Scott & Wade, 1969; Caine *et al.*, 1975), bromocriptine (Van Poppel *et al.*, 1987), 5-alpha-reductase inhibitors (Orlowski & Clark, 1988) and, more recently, laser-induced prostatectomy (Kabalin, 1993). The objective benefits of such treatments remain to be established and most may prove more costly in the long term than conventional TURP. However, all have the advantage that they avoid the risks associated with general or regional anaesthesia or have a more favourable haemodynamic profile due to reduced operative blood loss. They may thus be considered appropriate in the high-risk patient for whom established techniques are considered unsuitable.

Another alternative to conventional anaesthesia is TURP performed under local anaesthetic infiltration with or without sedation. Such a technique has been described by several authors (Moffat, 1977; Orandi, 1984; Sinha *et al.*, 1986; Loughlin *et al.*, 1987; Sarramon *et al.*, 1987). Most of these reports have been brief, anecdotal and lacking in objective evidence. Our own operating technique has been recently changed to one which employs sedation plus local anaesthesia — sedoanalgesia (Birch *et al.*, 1989). This has been shown to be safe, well tolerated and suitable for a wide range of patients independent of their age or level of fitness.

Local anaesthesia

There can be little doubt that procedures performed under local anaesthesia are inherently safer than those performed under general or regional anaesthesia (Shane, 1982; Coplans & Green, 1983; Hempenstall *et al.*, 1986). Patients also prefer them (Rodrigo & Clark, 1986; Rassam & Thomas, 1989; Birch *et al.*, 1990). Until recently, lower tract local anaesthesia was limited to the topical application of lignocaine to the urethra. However, there have recently been significant advances in the development of new local anaesthetic delivery systems. Thus the endoscopic needle described originally by Engberg *et al.* (1983) and Orandi (1984) and later modified by Miller *et al.* (1987) (Fig. 10.1) has, for the first time, allowed local anaesthetic infiltration of lower tract structures under direct vision. These needles have been designed specifically for endoscopic use and there are now few endoscopic procedures, including TURP, which cannot be performed under local anaesthesia.

Sedation

It is true to say that most endoscopic procedures can be performed under local anaesthesia alone. Indeed, many early cystoscopies were performed in exactly this way. However, such techniques fail to take account of the anxiety of patients undergoing even minor surgery (Birch *et al.*, 1993; Fig. 10.2). Even with adequate analgesia such procedures may be embarrassing or unpleasant. The use of a sedative

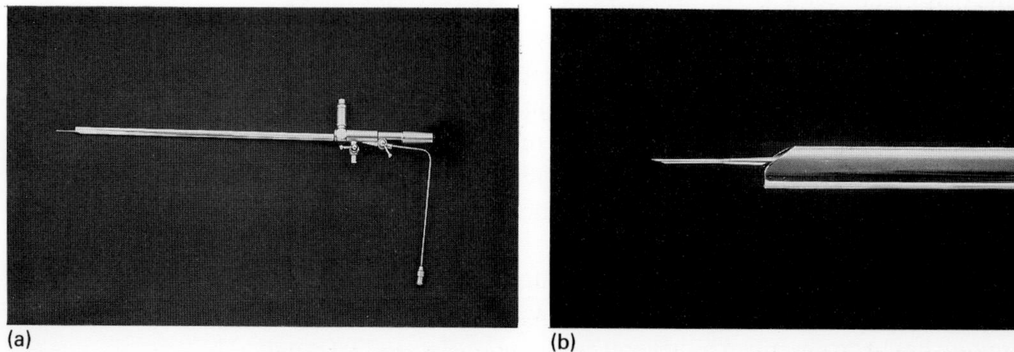

(a) (b)

Fig. 10.1. Endoneedle shown exiting from the instrument channel of the Integrated Cystoscope. (a) Whole view. (b) Close-up of instrument tip.

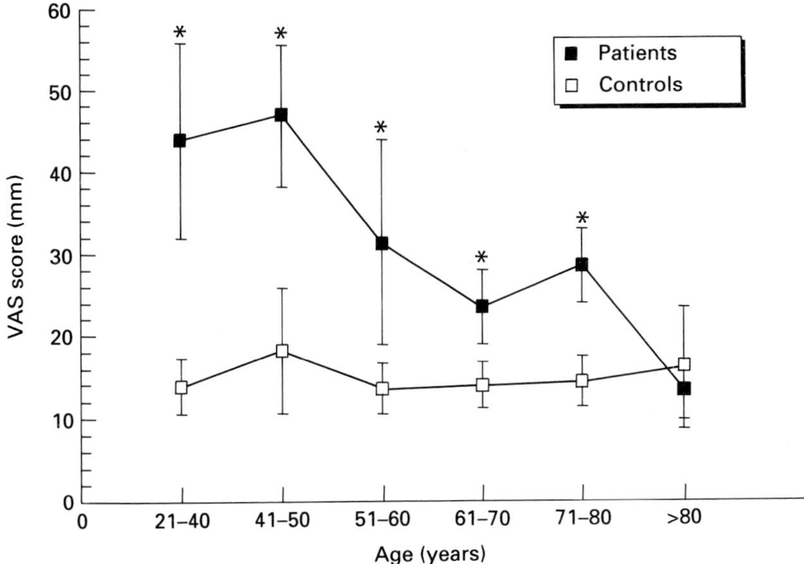

Fig. 10.2. Graph of anxiety (mm on a visual analogue scale) vs. age (years) for patients undergoing day-case cystoscopy and controls (matched for previous operative experience). All values expressed as mean ± 1 SEM. (* = $P < 0.05$, student's *t*-test, one-tailed.)

to supplement such procedures can significantly improve patient tolerance of surgery where this is to be performed under local anaesthesia (Hoare & Hawkins, 1976; Hanno & Wein, 1983). In this respect benzodiazepines prove both safe and effective. The most frequently used agents in this class of drugs are diazepam (Valium, Roche) and midazolam (Hypnovel, Roche). Midazolam, with its shorter duration of action, lack of tissue irritation, more profound anterograde amnesia and excellent uptake following intramuscular administration offers significant advantages over diazepam.

In our own practice of local anaesthetic TURP, midazolam is used as a pre-medication given by intramuscular injection 30 minutes preoperatively. This ensures that a calm, relaxed, sedated patient arrives in theatre ready for operation. Post-operatively, residual sedation may be reversed using the specific benzodiazepine antagonist flumazenil (see below).

Sedoanalgesia

The minimally invasive endoscopic techniques now available for urological surgery mean that the anaesthetic techniques used routinely for conventional surgical procedures are no longer appropriate. Sedoanalgesic techniques have been developed as a direct response to this. The term sedoanalgesia was chosen to give equal emphasis to the two components of this technique, namely sedation (using midazolam) and analgesia (using the local anaesthetics lignocaine and bupivicaine).

This concept of using sedation to supplement local anaesthetic procedures is not new (Scamman *et al.*, 1985; Goerig *et al.*, 1989). However, sedoanalgesia exploits advances in instrument technology, local anaesthetic delivery systems and drug research which serve to give it a distinctive nature (Miller *et al.*, 1990). The remainder of this chapter details the technique which allows TURP to be performed successfully under sedoanalgesia.

Operative technique

Pre-medication

Twenty to thirty minutes prior to surgery a pre-medication is administered. For this purpose midazolam is given by intramuscular injection into the deltoid, vastus lateralis or gluteal muscles. The dose used depends on the weight, age and overall fitness of the patient. In general, the dose of midazolam we use is 5–7.5 mg for those patients under 70 kg and 7.5–10 mg for heavier patients. This is equivalent to 0.1–0.12 mg/kg. For younger, anxious patients, the upper limit of this range is appropriate but in the unfit, elderly patient increased sensitivity to the effects of benzodiazepines demands an appropriate dosage reduction (30–50%). Table 10.1 gives a guide to dosage selection.

Ten to fifteen minutes after the administration of midazolam the urethra is anaesthetized using 2% lignocaine (20 g) applied topically as a gel and massaged along the length of the penis. A penile clamp is used to retain the gel within the urethra.

In this fashion, the patient is rendered calm and sedated prior to transfer to the operating theatre. The amnesic effect of the midazolam also ensures that the majority of patients have no recall for either the application of the topical anaesthetic and, in many cases, the operation itself.

Table 10.1. Premedication: guide to midazolam (i.m.) dosage

	ASA I and II		ASA III and IV	
Age range (years)	Dose (mg/kg)	Maximum (mg)	Dose (mg/kg)	Maximum (mg)
<55	0.10	10	0.05	5
56–65	0.08	7	0.04	4
66–75	0.06	5	0.03	3
>75	0.05	3	0.03	2

General

In order to reduce levels of sensory stimulation the ambient lighting level in theatre is lowered and noise kept to a minimum. Background music also proves helpful in this respect. Following arrival in theatre a further 20 g of 2% lignocaine gel is administered urethrally. This manoeuvre serves to increase the chances of successful topical anaesthesia of the posterior urethra. In our experience if the patient complains of discomfort at this stage during the administration of the lignocaine gel then the chances of successful local anaesthetic TURP are decreased considerably and supplemental intravenous analgesia (e.g. fentanyl) may be required.

As a routine measure, all patients receive supplemental oxygen by means of nasal cannulae and are monitored using a pulse oximeter (to guard against oxygen desaturation). Continuous ECG display and automatic blood pressure monitoring (Dinamap, Critiron, USA) are also employed routinely. These monitoring techniques are of particular importance in unfit patients who, on physical examination, fall in the American Society of Anesthesiologists (ASA) grades III and IV (ASA, 1963). Such patients tolerate hypoxaemia poorly. Intravenous access by means of a forearm cannula is established and a normal saline infusion commenced.

Peri-operatively the patient must be monitored by anaesthetic colleagues. A nurse should be delegated to speak to and reassure the patient throughout the procedure.

Those patients who are still anxious when they arrive in theatre may require supplemental intravenous midazolam before the procedure begins. This should be given slowly, in increments of 1 mg, the dose being titrated against clinical effect. In general, 1–3 mg is adequate.

Preliminary cystoscopy and local anaesthetic injection

Immediately before cystoscopy it is helpful to flush the urethra with 5–10 ml of saline or 1% lignocaine plain so as to clear it of lignocaine gel and improve visibility. Cystoscopy is then carried out using the Integrated Cystoscope (GU Manufacturing, UK) (Miller *et al.*, 1987) with the patient in the extended lithotomy position. Once intravesical pathology has been excluded local anaesthetic injection can be performed. Anaesthesia of the bladder neck and prostate is achieved by the injection of 1% lignocaine plain (10 ml) subtrigonally to either side of the ureteric orifices as shown in Fig. 10.3(a). Further injections (Fig. 10.3(a)) of a haemostatic local anaesthetic mixture (10 ml) are carried out in the bladder neck (at each of four quadrants, i.e. 5, 7, 2 and 10 o'clock) and prostate (laterally into each lobe and into the floor just proximal to the veru). It is important that the prostatic injections should be deep, out towards the capsule (Fig. 10.3(b)). The

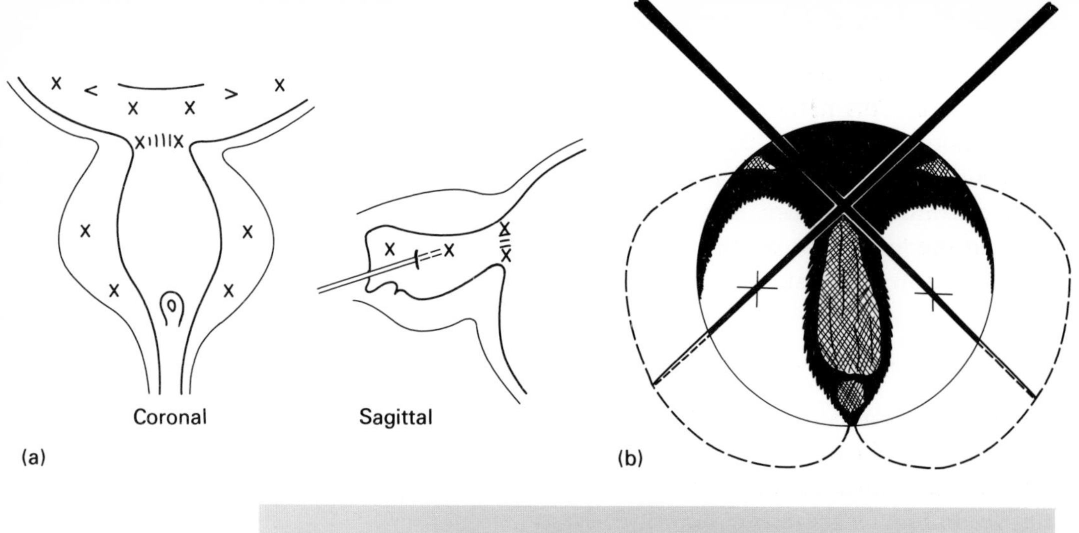

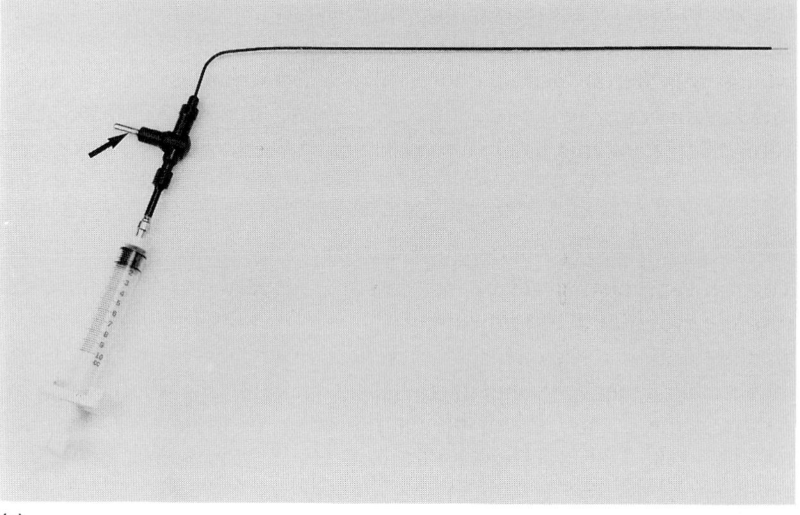

Fig. 10.3. (a) Injection sites in trigone, bladder neck and prostate. (b) Depth of prostatic injection (dotted outline = capsule). (c) Electrotest needle (diathermy coupling arrowed).

haemostatic local anaesthetic referred to above consists of 5 ml of 1% lignocaine plain mixed with 5 ml of 1% lignocaine with adrenaline 1 in 200 000. If further local anaesthesia is required 10–20 ml of 1% lignocaine plain suffices. An insulated endoscopic needle — the Birch–Miller Electrotest needle (Birch & Miller, 1991) — is also available for endoscopic local anaesthetic injection. This needle may be connected to a diathermy source to enable testing of injected areas prior to resection so as to ensure that adequate analgesia has been achieved (Fig. 10.3(c)).

Urethral dilatation and prostatic resection

Following local anaesthetic injection the urethra is dilated to 26 Ch with sounds. This manoeuvre serves to overcome resistance due to contraction or spasm of the distal sphincter. A standard transurethral resection is then performed using a conventional 24 Ch continuous-flow resectoscope (Storz, c/o Rimmer Bros, UK). If resectoscopes without the facility for continuous flow are used care must be taken not to overfill the bladder.

Post-operative management

Residual sedation is reversed using the specific benzodiazepine antagonist flumazenil (Anexate, Roche, UK) in a dose of 0.5 mg given as an intravenous bolus. Vesical irrigation via a 22 Ch three-way catheter (Porges Dufour) is used routinely. Early catheter removal is advocated and catheters are removed on the first or second post-operative night, where possible, at around midnight (Feldstein & Benson, 1988). In this fashion most patients can be discharged within 48–72 hours of admission when this has been accomplished on the day of operation.

Patient selection

TURP under sedoanalgesia is best suited to prostates where the weight of resected material is estimated to be no more than 40 g. Whilst larger glands could be resected limitations are imposed by the length of time for which a patient may be reasonably expected to remain comfortable whilst in the extended lithotomy position.

Results

Over 150 patients have had prostatic resections performed under sedoanalgesia in our department to date.

Of the first 100 patients treated in this fashion 80 presented with symptoms of outflow obstruction and 20 with acute retention of urine. The average age, weight and ASA grades of these patients are shown in Table 10.2.

The average dose of intramuscular midazolam required to achieve adequate operative sedation was 6.6 mg (range 3–10 mg). The use of additional intravenous midazolam, as an intra-operative supplement, was required in just 10 patients (10%). The average dose used was 2.2 mg (range 1–4 mg).

Operative details and flow rates (pre- and post-operative) are detailed in Tables 10.3 and 10.4 respectively.

Average haemoglobin concentrations fell from 13.8 g/dl pre-operatively to 12.1 g/dl post-operatively. Seven patients received a blood transfusion.

Table 10.2. Patient demography

Number	100
Age	Average 68.2 years (Range 44–94 years)
Weight	Average 72.9 kg (Range 57–104 kg)
ASA Grade I	3
II	51
III	42
IV	4

Table 10.3. Operative details

Duration
Average 23.6 min (range 15–35 min)

Resected weight
Average 11.1 g (range 2–35 g), 20% > 15 g

Histology
Benign: 94
Malignant: 6

Haemoglobin (g/dl)
Pre-op.: average 13.8 (range 9.2–17.4)
Post-op.: average 12.1 (range 7.7–16.4)

Transfusion
7 patients

Table 10.4. Flow rates

Patient group	Number	Status	Flow rate (ml/s)
Outflow obstruction	80	Pre-operative Post-operative	8.5 (range 2–20) 23.9 (range 3–35)
Acute retention	20	Post-operative	21.0 (range 12–29)

Standard (100 mm) visual analogue scales (where 0 = no pain and 100 = maximal pain) were used to rate patient discomfort. These showed that discomfort for the procedure was + 10 (range 0–45) as scored by the patients and + 9 (range 0–37) as rated by an independent observer. By way of comparison, pain related to the pre-operative injection of midazolam was + 3 (range 0–12). However, it should be noted that as resection nears completion pericapsular manipulations may cause some discomfort. In so far as this prevents capsular perforation such an occurrence is to be regarded as an additional safety feature of the technique.

No complications related to the use of midazolam and flumazenil have been noted to date. In particular, there have been no reports of post-operative anxiety or arousal. One patient died post-operatively from a pulmonary embolus confirmed at autopsy.

It can be inferred from the above that TURP performed under sedoanalgesia is safe, well tolerated and effective.

Local anaesthetic TURP: place in urological practice

Whilst many early endoscopic resections may have been performed under local anaesthesia, it was not until Moffatt's paper in 1977 that a local anaesthetic technique adapted specifically for endoscopic surgery was formally described. Local anaesthetic infiltration of the prostate was initially performed by blind transperineal injection. Suprapubic prostate injection under endoscopic control has also been described (Hak-Hagir, 1989). The accuracy of injection techniques improved with the advent of the first needles designed specifically for endoscopic use (Engberg *et al.*, 1983; Orandi, 1984). These needles could be passed along the instrument channel of a conventional 24 Ch resectoscope and used for local anaesthetic injection under direct vision. The use of smaller, less traumatic instruments together with modifications of these needles has been reported by other authors (Miller *et al.*, 1987).

Sedation alone: disadvantages

The possibility that the above procedures could be performed without local anaesthesia using sedation alone can be refuted by the experience of those endoscopists who have attempted resection where the local anaesthetic block has been less than adequate. Further proof comes from a report of prostatic resection under sedation alone (Lightwardt & Girgis, 1985). In this study 65 patients underwent TURP. Most experienced discomfort and the majority (58/65) required supplementation with intravenous fentanyl or ketamine.

Local anaesthesia alone: the role of sedation

Can these same procedures be performed under local anaesthesia alone? The answer is 'yes' but there is no doubt that the use of sedation to supplement local anaesthesia increases patient tolerance significantly (Hoare & Hawkins, 1976; Hanno & Wein, 1983). Midazolam, unlike diazepam, exhibits excellent uptake following intramuscular injection. This property of midazolam allows it to be used effectively for pre-medication. It should be noted that benzodiazepines do not have any direct analgesic activity. Pain relief must be achieved by the use of a good local anaesthetic block. It is unacceptable merely to sedate patients so heavily that they have no recall of intraoperative pain. The surgeon should be seeking, primarily, to exploit the anxiolytic properties of these drugs. Any amnesic action should be seen as a useful additional component of drug activity, not an excuse to ablate the memory for an otherwise unacceptable procedure.

General and regional anaesthesia: safety of sedoanalgesia

The majority of patients requiring prostatic surgery are suitable for general or regional anaesthesia. This fact is advanced by some as obviating the need for local anaesthetic resection. However, conventional techniques are not without related morbidity and mortality and may be unsuitable for patients with significant cardiopulmonary disease. They may also be technically difficult, time-consuming and associated with a greater number of complications.

In our own practice of TURP under sedoanalgesia, operation was initially restricted to those patients unfit for conventional anaesthetic techniques. However, the success of such surgery quickly led to its adoption as the procedure of choice for healthier patients. This was a logical step and proved equally successful. In our unit, all patients with glands less than 40 g are now treated in this fashion. A similar experience was reported by Sinha *et al.* (1986).

TURP under sedoanalgesia: application

The 40 g upper limit selected for local anaesthetic TURP has not been imposed for technical reasons. Rather, the limiting factor is the amount of time for which the conscious patient can be reasonably expected to stay in the lithotomy position before muscular discomfort supervenes. Even so, given recent data relating to TURP (Mebust *et al.*, 1989), the majority (approximately 60%) of all prostates presenting for surgery could be treated in this way.

Flumazenil

The use of the specific benzodiazepine antagonist flumazenil postoperatively will reverse residual sedation and ensure an alert, cooperative patient (Birch *et al.*, 1990). This allows for early ambulation and thereby serves to minimize potential thrombo-embolic and pulmonary problems related to surgery. The cost of flumazenil is thus offset by the reduction in theatre, nursing and recovery time that results from the above (Birch *et al.*, 1988).

TURP under sedoanalgesia: advantages

Sedoanalgesia preserves detrusor function and sphincter co-ordination (unlike regional blocks) whilst at the same time allowing virtually immediate ambulation with resumption of a normal fluid and solid diet (unlike general anaesthesia). The possibilities for day-case surgery (Perez, 1985; Moffat, 1987) are thereby enhanced.

Summary

Our experience and the results of this study show that local anaesthetic TURP is safe, effective, well tolerated and suitable for all patients with glands less than 40 g who require TURP. The benefits of early ambulation and bladder control then enable the surgeon to exploit the possibilities for reduced post-operative stay where this is considered desirable.

References

American Society of Anesthesiologists (ASA) (1963) Editorial: New classification of physical status. *Anesthesiology*, **24**, 111.

Angell J.C. (1969) Treatment of benign prostatic hyperplasia by phenol injection. *Br. J. Urol.*, **41**, 735–8.

Birch B.R.P. & Miller R.A. (1991) The Birch–Miller Electrotest needle: An aid to local anaesthetic endoscopic surgery. *Urology*, **38**, 64–5.

Birch B.R.P., Anson K.M., Clifford E. & Miller R.A. (1988) Use of hospital beds. *Br. Med. J.*, **297**, 1404–5.

Birch B.R.P., Anson K.M., Gelister J. & Miller R.A. (1989) Sedoanalgesia in urology: technique, applications and impact. *World J. Urol.*, **7**, 162–5.

Birch B.R.P., Anson K.M., Gelister J., Parker C. & Miller R.A. (1990) The role of midazolam and flumazenil in urology. *Acta Anaesthesiol. Scand.*, **32** (Suppl. 19), 25–32.

Birch B.R.P., Chakraborty R. & Miller R.A. (1993) Anxiety levels in patients undergoing local anaesthetic day-case cystoscopy. *J. One-Day Surg.*, **3**, 15–17.

Caine M., Perlberg S. & Gordon R. (1975) The treatment of benign prostatic hypertrophy with flutamide (SCH 13521): a placebo controlled study. *J. Urol.*, **114**, 564–8.

Caine M., Perlberg S. & Meretyk S. (1978) A placebo controlled double blind study of the effect of phenoxybenzamine in benign prostatic obstruction. *Br. J. Urol.*, **50**, 551–4.

Coplans M.P. & Green R.A. (1983) Mortality and morbidity studies. In: Coplans M.P. & Green R.A. (eds) *Anaesthesia and Sedation in Dentistry*. Monographs in Anaesthesiology (Vol. 12), pp. 131–47. Elsevier, Amsterdam.

Engberg A., Spanberg A. & Urnes T. (1983) Transurethral resection of bladder tumours under local anaesthesia. *Urology*, **22**, 385–7.

Fabian K.M. (1978) Der interprostatische 'partielle katheter' (Urologische Spirale) II. *Urologie (A)*, **23**, 229–33.

Feldstein M.S. & Benson N.A. (1988) Early catheter removal and reduced length of hospital stay following transurethral prostatectomy: A retrospective analysis of 100 consecutive patients. *J. Urol.*, **140**, 532–4.

Ferrie B.G. & Paterson P.J. (1987) Phenoxybenzamine in prostatic hypertrophy. A double blind study. *Br. J. Urol.*, **59**, 63–5.

Gill K.P., Machan L.S., Allison D.J. & Williams G. (1989) Bladder outflow tract obstruction and urinary retention from benign prostatic hypertrophy treated by balloon dilatation. *Br. J. Urol.*, **64**, 618–22.

Goerig M., Filos K. & Beck H. (1989) Georg Perthes (1869–1927): A pioneer of local anaesthesia by blocking peripheral nerves with the use of electrical stimulation. *Royal Society of Medicine, International Congress and Symposium Series*, **134**, 551–8.

Graverson P.H., Gasser T.C., Wasson J.H., Hinman F. Jr. & Bruskewitz R.C. (1989) Controversies about indications for transurethral resection of the prostate. *J. Urol.*, **141**, 475–81.

Hak-Hagir A. (1989) Transurethral electroresection of a vesical cervix obstruction under local anaesthesia. Seventh World Congress of Endourology and ESWL, Kyoto, Japan, Abstract V2-1, p. 262.

Hanno P.M. & Wein A.J. (1983) Anesthetic techniques for cystoscopy in men. *J. Urol.*, **130**, 1070–2.

Hempenstall P.D., Campbell J.P.S., Bajurnow A.T., Reade P.C., McGrath B. & Harrison L.C. (1986) Cardiovascular, biochemical and hormonal responses to intravenous sedation with local analgesia versus general anaesthesia in patients undergoing oral surgery. *J. Oral Maxillofac. Surg.*, **44**, 441–6.

Hoare A.M. & Hawkins C.F. (1976) Upper gastrointestinal endoscopy with and without sedation: patients' opinions. *Br. Med. J.*, **ii**, 20.

Kabalin J.N. (1993) Laser prostatectomy performed with a right angle firing neodymium:YAG laser at 40 watts power. *J. Urol.*, **150**, 95–9.

Keane P.F., Timoney A.G., Kiely E., Williams G. & Stamp G. (1988) Response of the benign hypertrophied prostate to treatment with an LHRH analogue. *Br. J. Urol.*, **62**, 163–5.

Kirby R.S., Coppinger S.W.C., Corcoran M.O., Chapple C.R., Flannigan M. & Milroy E.J.G. (1987) Prazosin in the treatment of prostatic obstruction. A placebo controlled study. *Br. J. Urol.*, **60**, 136–42.

Lightwardt J.R. & Girgis S. (1985) Transurethral resection of prostate with intravenous sedation. *Urology*, **26**, 112–13.

Lindner A., Golomb J., Siegel Y. & Lev A. (1987) Local hyperthermia of the prostate gland for the treatment of benign prostatic hypertrophy and urinary retention. A preliminary report. *Br. J. Urol.*, **60**, 567–71.

Loughlin K.R., Yalla S.V., Belldegrun A. & Bernstein G.T. (1987) Transurethral incisions and resections under local anaesthesia. *Br. J. Urol.*, **60**, 185.

Mebust W.K., Holtgrewe H.L., Cockett A.T.K. & Peters P.C. (1989) Transurethral prostatectomy: Intermediate and post-operative complications. A cooperative study of 13 participating institutions evaluating 3885 patients. *J. Urol.*, **141**, 243–7.

Miller R.A., Coptcoat M.J., Parry J., Dawkins G. & Wickham J.E.A. (1987) The Integrated Cystoscope: An alternative to conventional and fibreoptic cystoscopy. *Br. J. Urol.*, **60**, 128–31.

Miller R.A., Birch B.R.P., Anson K.M., Bell J., Gelister J. & Grant D. (1990) The impact of minimally invasive surgery and sedoanalgesia on urological practice. *Postgrad. Med. J.*, (Suppl. 1), S72–S76.

Milroy E.J.G., Chapple C.R., Eldin A. & Wallsten H. (1989) A new stent for the treatment of urethral strictures. Preliminary report. *Br. J. Urol.*, **63**, 392–6.

Moffat, N.A. (1977) Transurethral prostatic resections under local anaesthesia. *J. Urol.*, **118**, 607–8.

Moffat N.A. (1987) Transurethral resection of prostate and bladder tumours. *Urol. Clin. N. Amer.*, **14**(1), 115–19.

Orandi A. (1984) Urological endoscopic surgery under local anaesthesia: A cost reducing idea. *J. Urol.*, **132**, 1146–7.

Orlowski J. & Clark A.F. (1988) Effect of a 4-methyl-4-aza steroid on androgen metabolism by rat ventral prostate epithelial and stromal cell cultures: Selective inhibition of 5-alpha-reductase activity. *The Prostate*, **13**, 289–97.

Perez J.A. (1985) Outpatient transurethral resection of the prostate. In: Kaye K.W. (ed.) *Outpatient Urologic Surgery*, Chapter 15, p. 120 *et seq*. Lea & Febiger, Philadelphia.

Rassam S. & Thomas H.F. (1989) Local anaesthesia for cataract surgery. *Lancet*, **i**, 110–11.

Rodrigo M.C. & Clark R.N.W. (1986) A study of intravenous sedation with diazepam and midazolam for dentistry in Hong Kong Chinese. *Anaesth. Intens. Care*, **14**, 404–11.

Sarramon J.P., Elman B. & Rischmann P. (1987) Endoscopic surgery under local anaesthesia. *Eur. Urol.*, **13**, 274–5.

Scamman F.L., Klein S.L. & Choi W.W. (1985) Conscious sedation for procedures under local or topical anaesthesia. *Ann. Otol. Rhinol. Laryngol.*, **94**, 21–4.

Scott W.W. & Wade J.C. (1969) Medical treatment of benign nodular prostatic hyperplasia with cyproterone acetate. *J. Urol.*, **101**, 81–5.

Servadio C., Leib Z. & Lev A. (1987) Diseases of prostate treated by local microwave hyperthermia. *Urology*, **30**, 97–9.

Shafik A. (1988) Closed prostatic commissurotomy. An endoscopic technique for the treatment of benign prostatic hypertrophy. *Br. J. Urol.*, **62**, 431–3.

Shane S.M. (1982) Conscious sedation and behavioural modification with local standby anaesthesia for ophthalmologic surgery. *Ophthalmic Surg.*, **13**, 50–2.

Sinha B., Haikel G., Lange P.H., Moon T.D. & Narayan P. (1986) Transurethral resection of the prostate with local anaesthesia in 100 patients. *J. Urol.*, **135**, 719–21.

Van Poppel H., Boeckx G., Westelinck K.J., Vereecken R.L. & Baert L. (1987) The efficacy of bromocriptine in benign prostatic hypertrophy. A double blind study. *Br. J. Urol.*, **60**, 150–2.

Wei X.Y. & Zhou X.M. (1987) 5-Fluorouracil (5-FU) in the treatment of prostatic hyperplasia. *Urol. Res.*, **15**, 35–7.

Wyatt M.G., Stower M.J., Smith P.J.B. & Roberts J.B.M. (1989) Prostatectomy in the over 80-year-old. *Br. J. Urol.*, **64**, 417–19.

11 Blood loss in transurethral surgery

S.W.V. COPPINGER AND C. HUDD

'I don't need to measure blood loss to know when my patient is bleeding' is an all too familiar cry from the experienced urologist. But how appropriate is it? Certainly, s/he has a good idea when significant loss is occurring, but quantifying it is another matter. Furthermore, the resectionist and anaesthetist in training may find it is easy to lose track and find the patient's circulation compromised. Unfortunately, the predominantly elderly patients who undergo transurethral resection of the prostate (TURP) are often treated with various medications which mask or delay the classical physiological response to bleeding, and signs of excessive blood loss occur at a stage at which it is poorly tolerated.

Gatch and Little, in 1924, drew attention to the blood loss which occurs in large operations and Pilcher and Sheard related this to transurethral surgery in 1937. In 1941 Nesbit & Conger studied 100 transurethral resections of the prostate, two-thirds of which were carried out by residents. Blood loss was measured calorimetrically at the end of the procedure by matching acid haematin precipitated from haemoglobin against known standard solutions. Average blood loss was 169 ml but about half of the resections were small glands or 'median bars'. Twenty-two per cent of the resections were over 35 g and these lost in excess of 250 ml. The authors believed that 'total blood loss' which included post-operative loss 'approximated twice the operative blood loss'. Interestingly, when this question was addressed in 1982 by Sleight he also concluded that blood lost in the 3 post-operative days was almost the same as that lost during the operation. Nesbit & Conger (1941) were also aware of the value in measuring blood loss during the procedure and attempted to quantify this by a series of complex manoeuvres followed by comparison against standard solutions.

The accurate measurement of blood loss during endoscopic resection has never been easy and most authors have relied on an estimate of blood loss at the end of the procedure. Methods of determination have included photoelectric, radioactive red-cell tagging, Evans blue determinations, change in conductivity and, mostly calorimetric estimations (Rives & Latchem, 1945; LeVeen & Rubricus, 1958; Litin & Emmett, 1959; Desmond, 1973). More recently a variety of more sophisticated methods have been used to estimate blood loss and range from haemoglobin extraction techniques, dye dilution, indicator dilution (using potassium ions as an intrinsic indicator) and latterly photometric techniques using single-wavelength photometry (Jansen *et al.*, 1978; Freedman *et al.*, 1985). Sources of error using haemoglobin extraction dilution techniques include error due to dilution of the known volume of water by the unknown volume of blood, inadequate destruction of blood clot, incomplete lysis of clot, inaccurate measurement of large volumes, errors associated with determination of haemoglobin and errors associated with variability of the haemoglobin of the shed blood. The latter can be due to haemodilution as a result of the physiological response to blood loss or fluid absorption, anaesthesia, intravenous infusion or blood transfusion (Bond, 1969). Some of these problems were addressed by modifications introduced by Lyrddal & Neidhardt (1984) who prevented clot formation by mechanical and chemical means. Hahn (1987) studied the influence of variations in blood haemoglobin concentration on the calculation of blood loss and volumetric irrigating fluid balance during TURP and concluded that blood loss was greater the later the blood haemoglobin was determined because loss of plasma was underestimated. He introduced a haemodilution factor to correct for this while accepting that, ideally, repeated sampling should be performed.

A method which reliably measures blood loss at any given time during the procedure would clearly be a major advance in establishing which patients have suffered sufficient loss to justify transfusion prior to developing the signs of blood loss. In collaboration with the Divisions of Bioengineering and Anaesthesia at Northwick Park Hospital and the Clinical Research Centre, we have been using an apparatus which measures total blood content in the blood–irrigant mixture (Hudd *et al.*, 1989). Blood loss is then calculated using the formula:

$$\frac{\text{Volume of blood–irrigant mixture} \times \text{mixture Hb}}{\text{Patient's Hb}}$$

The apparatus is depicted in Fig. 11.1. It consists of a bath into which the strained blood–irrigant mixture is collected by the scrub nurse. The bath rests on a set of scales attached to an electronic strain gauge. The bath weight is tared, and the contents weighed. Assuming a density of 1, the weight equates to the volume and this is entered into an electronic multiplier. The mixed blood–irrigant solution is circulated through a loop of tubing by a pump. A side arm of the loop is connected to a small peristaltic pump which, on demand, draws a sample from the loop through a photometric cell. This uses a green and a red light source, red being the reference and green the measuring wavelength. The optical density is the difference between the two wavelengths, and equates to the haemoglobin content.

On initiation of the cycle the system automatically zeros on the

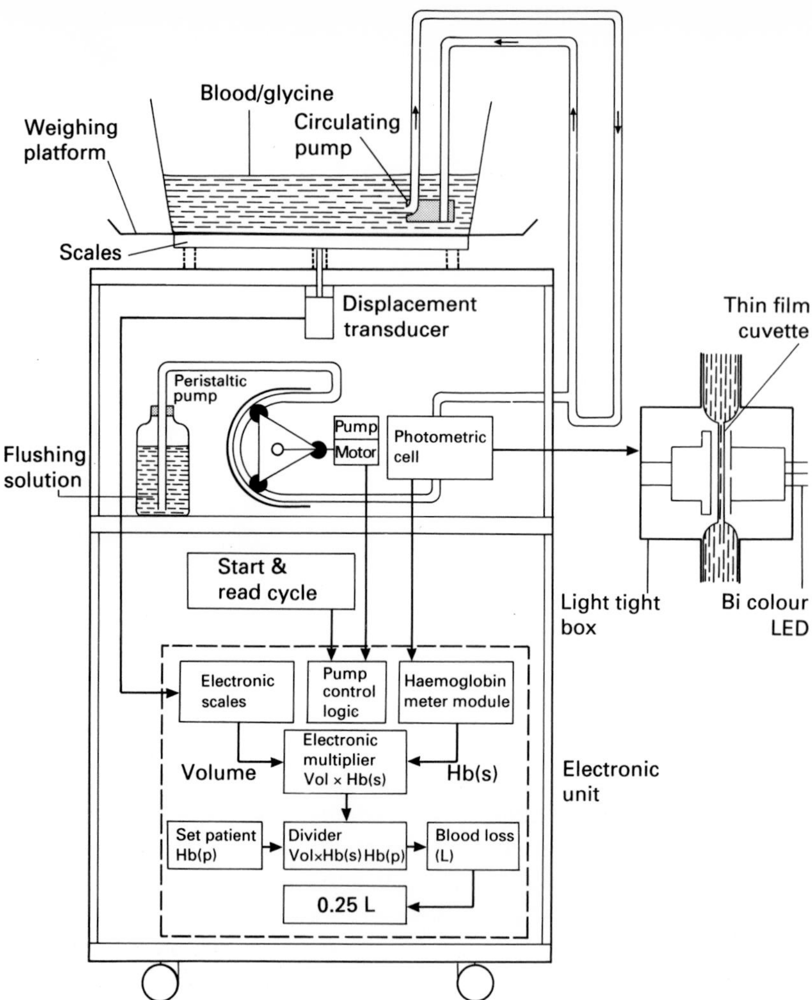

Fig. 11.1. Apparatus for measuring total blood content in the blood–irrigant mixture.

clear flushing solution in the photometric cell. The pump then aspirates a sample of the mixture from the loop and measures the optical density. The pump then reverses, replacing the sample with clear flushing solution. The optical density, expressed as haemoglobin, is entered into the electronic multiplier which multiplies this value by the volume (i.e. weight) of the mixture obtained from the strain gauge. It then divides this number by the patient's pre-operative haemoglobin level which is entered manually at the beginning of the procedure. On demand, a 'read' cycle is initiated, at the end of which the shed blood volume is displayed digitally using a liquid crystal display.

This technique has been evaluated in the clinical setting with most of the procedures being carried out by one surgeon. The decision whether to use general or regional anaesthesia was left to the anaes-

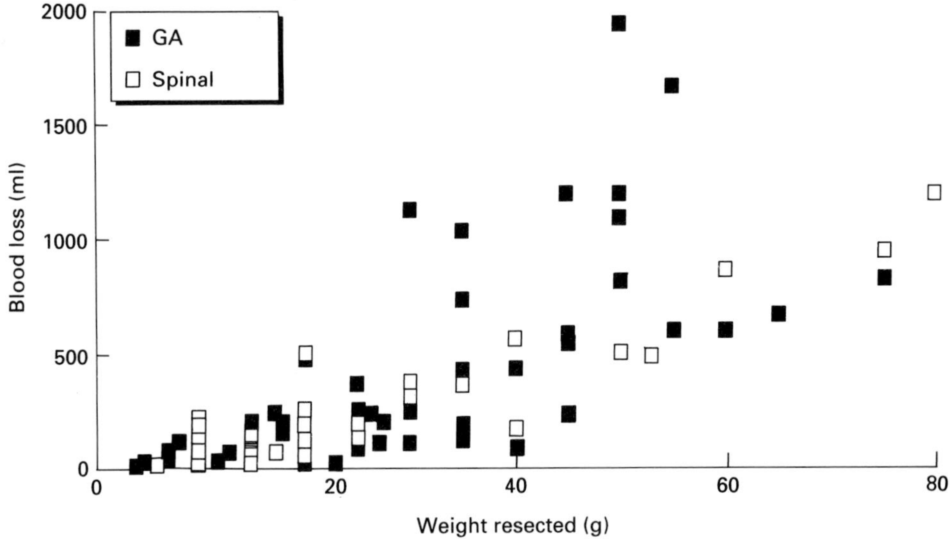

Fig. 11.2. Relationship between tissue resected and blood loss.

thetist and was based on clinical needs or personal preference. One hundred and thirty-one patients were studied. Eleven patients in whom data were incomplete were excluded leaving 119 patients for evaluation, 82 receiving general and 37 regional anaesthesia. The results are depicted in Table 11.1 and Fig. 11.2.

There is no significant difference between general and spinal anaesthetic groups in all the parameters measured. It is, however, interesting to note that blood loss was lower in the regional anaesthesia group and that this was not related to a drop in blood pressure. Indeed, blood pressure was higher in the regional anaesthesia group, a finding one might not expect. It is, however, consistent with our previous and other studies and is discussed later. There is a relationship between

Table 11.1. Comparison of patients undergoing TURP under general or spinal anaesthesia*

	Hb	BP	Duration	Wt resected (g)
GA	14.0 ± .2	116 ± 2	36 ± 2	27 ± 2
Spinal	14.3 ± .3	133 ± 3	37 ± 2	25 ± 3
	Blood loss (ml)	**Loss/g (ml/g)**	**Loss/min (ml/min)**	**Wt/min (g/min)**
GA	312 ± 42	9.7 ± 0.9	7.2 ± 0.8	0.7 ± 0.1
spinal 2	257 ± 45	9.2 ± 0.9	6.2 ± 0.8	0.7 ± 0.1

* Means ± SEM.

tissue resected and blood loss (GA $r = 0.71$, $P < 0.001$; spinal $r = 0.92$, $P < 0.001$). Irrespective of mode of anaesthesia, there is no correlation between blood pressure and rate of blood loss or total blood loss.

This direct, on-demand, dual-wavelength photometric method has shown itself to be easy to use, rapid, and reliable. The technique of dual-wavelength photometry automatically compensates for optical scatter caused by debris, thus measuring only the haemoglobin in the blood–irrigant mixture. Clot formation is prevented by the addition of heparin to the collecting bath. These features thus obviate many of the criticisms mentioned earlier. The accuracy of the apparatus was validated by using known dilutions of whole blood and comparing the measurements made by the apparatus with those obtained using standard laboratory equipment. One criticism mentioned before is that of haemodilution during the procedure. This has been addressed in a small study. Although the discrepancy, which averaged 67 ml, is small, it is recommended that in the trial setting the patient's haemoglobin should be entered at induction of anaesthesia and at the end of each full collecting bath.

This is an uncontrolled series of patients with no definite isolation of variables such as individual operator or anaesthetist, type of anaesthesia and so on. Nevertheless, both surgeons and anaesthetists have found the ease of blood loss estimation useful. We compared visual estimates of blood loss with actual blood loss during TURP and found that even experienced urologists overestimated blood loss up to a level of 200 ml and underestimated thereafter. Interestingly, with experience these figures improved until blood loss exceeded 500 ml.

In considering the topic of blood loss during transurethral prostatectomy there are a number of factors which are worthy of mention. There is a relationship to size which tends to increase exponentially as the size increases. This can also be related to length of resection, allowing blood loss to be expressed as loss per gram and loss per minute. Operator experience is certainly related to blood loss and it is wise for the budding urologist to exercise caution with larger glands.

The type of anaesthesia may be related to blood loss. Spinal or epidural anaesthesia is associated with less shedding of blood in some studies although this has not been necessarily confirmed by others (Abrams *et al.*, 1982; Nielsen *et al.*, 1987; Mackenzie, 1990). These findings were not related to changes in arterial blood pressure but the reduced loss is thought to be associated with a lack of rise in central venous pressure seen under general anaesthesia and possibly a reduced local prostatic venous complex pressure. Epidural anaesthesia reduces blood loss in retropubic prostatectomy (Hendolin & Alhava, 1982).

Post-prostatectomy bleeding has been attributed to the dissolution of clots by the action of urokinase normally present in urine and excess plasminogen activator produced as a result of surgical trauma. Epsilon-aminocaproic acid prevents this dissolution by inhibiting the activation of plasminogen by urokinase. A number of authors have sought to exploit this phenomenon and reduce post-TURP bleeding by systemic or intravesical administration. Early studies suggested that post-operative bleeding is reduced whereas others have failed to confirm these results (Vinnicombe & Shuttleworth, 1966; Smith *et al.*, 1984; Flanigan *et al.*, 1985; Sharifi *et al.*, 1986). Given orally, after removal of the catheter, the incidence of secondary haemorrhage was reduced with tranexamic acid (Miller *et al.*, 1980). Essentially, it seems that its early use has fallen into disrepute because of problems with indissoluble clot and its late use is still advocated by some. Fibrin adhesive (consisting of fibrinogen concentrate and thrombin, thus mimicking the last step in blood clotting) instilled at the conclusion of TURP has been shown to reduce post-operative blood loss, but has failed to gain popularity (Luke *et al.*, 1986).

There is no significant difference in blood loss, or glycine absorption, between continuous-flow and intermittent-flow transurethral resection (Stephenson *et al.*, 1980; Flechner & Williams, 1982). Warming the irrigating fluid has no effect on blood loss but does decrease patient heat loss and shivering (Heathcote & Dyer, 1986; Oszlanczi & Szabo, 1990). Endoscopic injection of ornithine-8-vasopressin into the prostate leads to a significant decrease in blood loss during TURP under general or spinal anaesthesia (Smart, 1984). The generalized vasoconstriction and hypertension associated with this technique have prevented its general use.

The use of prophylactic subcutaneous heparin in patients undergoing major surgery has been advocated for a number of years. However, its routine use in endoscopic surgery has not gained much support, presumably because of the low incidence of thrombotic sequelae. Various studies have been at odds as to the value of minidose heparin. It seems that minidose heparin does not affect blood loss, is safe in patients undergoing TURP and has a place in the patient at high risk of thrombosis or embolism (Bejjani *et al.*, 1983; Wilson *et al.*, 1988).

With improved cross-matching techniques it is usually sufficient to 'group and save serum' rather than 'cross-match' as was previously advocated. In reviewing the subject, Jenkins & Mintz (1981) put forward compelling medical and financial arguments in favour of a 'group and save' policy for the majority of patients. After all, the time taken to obtain blood in this situation is no different from that of asking for extra blood during a procedure. Those who are unconvinced could always take to measuring blood loss routinely!

In conclusion, visual estimates of blood loss are notoriously inaccurate and yet seem to be universally accepted. It is possible to measure blood loss during TURP more or less accurately and the reader must decide which is appropriate to his or her needs. At the end of the day there is a lot to be said for sound technique and a few minutes spent checking the bleeding during and at the conclusion of the procedure will be well rewarded.

Acknowledgements

We wish to gratefully acknowledge the help of Roger Colbeck, David Mee and David White in the carrying out of the studies at Northwick Park Hospital and Clinical Research Centre.

References

Abrams P.H., Shah P.J.R., Bryning K., Gaches C.G.C., Ashken M.H. & Green N.A. (1982) Blood loss during transurethral prostatectomy. *Anaesthesia*, **37**, 71–3.

Bejjani B.B., Chen D.C.P., Nolan N.G. & Edson M. (1983) Minidose heparin in transurethral prostatectomy. *Urology*, **22**, 251–4.

Bond A.G. (1969) Determination of operative blood loss. The sources of error and elimination of inaccuracy in the haemoglobin-dilution technique. *Anaesthesia*, **24**, 219–29.

Desmond J. (1973) A method of measuring blood loss during transurethral prostatic surgery. *J. Urol.*, **109**, 453–6.

Flanigan R.C., Butler K.M., O'Neal W., Rapp R.P., Casale A.J., Allen D.C. & McRoberts J.W. (1985) Comparison of epsilon aminocaproic acid and normal saline for postoperative bladder irrigation following transurethral resection of prostate. *Urology*, **26**, 227–8.

Flechner S.M. & Williams R.D. (1982) Continuous flow and conventional resectoscope methods in transurethral prostatectomy: comparative study. *J. Urol.*, **127**, 257.

Freedman M., van der Molen S.W. & Makings E. (1985) Blood loss measurement during transurethral resection of the prostate gland. *Br. J. Urol.*, **57**, 311–6.

Hahn R.G. (1987) Influence of variations in blood haemoglobin concentration on the calculation of blood loss and volumetric irrigating fluid balance during transurethral resection of the prostate. *Br. J. Anaesth.*, **59**, 1223–9.

Heathcote P.S. & Dyer P.M. (1986) The effect of warm irrigation on blood loss during transurethral prostatectomy under spinal anaesthesia. *Br. J. Urol.*, **58**, 669.

Hendolin H. & Alhava E. (1982) Effect of epidural versus general anaesthesia on peroperative blood loss during retropubic prostatectomy. *Int. Urol. Nephrol.*, **14**, 399–405.

Hudd C., Colbeck R., White D. *et al.* (1989) Measurement of blood loss during transurethral resection of the prostate. *J. Urol.*, **141** 4, 283.

Jansen H.J., Bersus O. & Johansson J.E. (1978) A simple photometric method for determination of blood loss during transurethral surgery. *Scand. J. Urol. Nephrol.*, **12**, 1–5.

Jenkins A.D. & Mintz P.D. (1981) Optimal blood use in genitourinary surgery. *J. Urol.*, **126**, 497–9.

LeVeen H.H. & Rubricus J.L. (1958) Continuous, automatic, electronic determinations of operative blood loss. *Surg. Gynec. Obst.*, **106**, 368–74.

Litin R.B. & Emmett J.L. (1959) Method for measuring blood loss during transurethral resection when nonhemolytic irrigation solutions are employed. *Proc. Mayo Clin.*, **34**, 158.

Luke M., Kvist E., Andersen F. & Hjortrup A. (1986) Reduction of postoperative bleeding after transurethral resection of the prostate by local instillation of fibrin adhesive (Beriplast). *Br. J. Urol.*, **58**, 672–5.

Lyrdal F. & Neidhardt F.O. (1984) Determination of blood loss during transurethral prostatic resection. Modification of a method. *Scand. J. Urol. Nephrol.*, **18**, 97–100.

Mackenzie A.R. (1990) Influence of anaesthesia on blood loss in transurethral prostatectomy. *Sct. Med. J.*, **35**, 14–16.

Miller R.A., May M.W., Hendry W.F., Whitfield H.N. & Wickham J.E.A. (1980) The prevention of secondary haemorrhage after prostatectomy: the value of antifibrinolytic therapy. *Br. J. Urol.*, **52**, 26–8.

Nesbit R.M. & Conger K.B. (1941) Studies of blood loss during transurethral prostatic resection. *J. Urol.*, **46**, 713–7.

Nielsen K.K., Andersen K., Asbjorn J., Vork F. & Ohrt-Nissen A. (1987) Blood loss in transurethral prostatectomy: epidural versus general anaesthesia. *Int. Urol. Nephrol.*, **19**, 287–92.

Oszlanczi J. & Szabo M. (1990) Measuring blood loss during transurethral resections. *Acta Chir. Hungarica*, **31**, 69–73.

Rives H.F. & Latchem C.W. (1945) A table for determination of blood loss during transurethral prostatic resection. *Proc. Staff Meet. Mayo Clin.*, **20**, 151–5.

Sharifi R., Lee M., Ray P., Millner S.N. & Dupont P.F. (1986) Safety and efficacy of intravesical aminocaproic acid for bleeding after transurethral resection of prostate. *Urology*, **27**, 214–9.

Sleight M.W. (1982) The effect of prophylactic subcutaneous heparin on blood loss during and after transurethral prostatectomy. *Br. J. Urol.*, **54**, 164–5.

Smart R.F. (1984) Endoscopic injection of the vasoconstrictor ornithine-8-vasopressin in transurethral resection. *Br. J. Urol.*, **56**, 191–7.

Smith R.B., Riach P. & Kaufman J.J. (1984) Epsilon aminocaproic acid and the control of post-prostatectomy bleeding: a prospective double-blind study. *J. Urol.*, **131**, 1093–5.

Stephenson T.O., Latto P., Bradley D., Hayward M. & Jones A. (1980) Comparison between continuous flow and intermittent flow transurethral resection in 40 patients presenting with acute retention. *Br. J. Urol.*, **52**, 523–5.

Vinnicombe J. & Shuttleworth K.E.D. (1966) Aminocaproic acid in the control of haemorrhage after prostatectomy: a controlled trial. *Lancet*, **1**, 230–2.

Wilson R.G., Smith D., Paton G., Gollock J.M. & Bremner D.N. (1988) Prophylactic subcutaneous heparin does not increase operative blood loss in transurethral resection of the prostate. *Br. J. Urol.*, **62**, 246–8.

12 Advances in laser therapy

T. McNICHOLAS

Introduction

The rapid development and improvement of new treatment methods and the endoscopic equipment with which to perform them allowed the enormous expansion of endoscopic urology. Since we are enthusiasts for new technology, particularly when relevant to endoscopic techniques, it is not surprising that urologists were among the first to apply the new method of delivering and applying energy that the introduction of clinically accessible laser units allowed.

There is a current upsurge of interest in non-surgical methods of treatment of benign prostatic enlargement at present. Whilst traditional transurethral resection of the prostate (TURP) is a difficult operation to beat in terms of immediate efficacy it does have complications and morbidity. There is a longer-term cloud hanging over TURP with regard to long-term cardiovascular side-effects (Roos *et al.*, 1989). Amongst the recent developments microwaves have caught the public attention but are not easily focused and usually involve several treatment visits. The early machines had no obvious histopathological effect on the prostate tissue and whilst later machines may cause tissue effects they are extremely expensive. Against this background there has been a reappraisal of the use of laser energy for prostatic therapy.

Although most available lasers have at some time been directed against prostatic tissue there are either major disadvantages to most, or a lack of efficacy, so that the neodymium–yttrium–aluminium–garnet (Nd–YAG) laser is the only practical laser of real interest at present. However, its position is unlikely to remain unchallenged and there are a range of other laser wavelength therapies approaching the end of the 'experimental' stage and nearing clinical evaluation for prostatic disease.

The theoretical basis for the laser (an acronym for 'light amplification by stimulated emission of radiation') was established by Einstein. However, its practical development did not occur until 1960. A laser is capable of generating an intense parallel beam of electromagnetic energy of a given wavelength. The primary characteristics of a laser beam are monochromatic light that can be transmitted and focused with precision and the light energy contained in the beam can be delivered with little loss of energy elsewhere.

Lasers differ primarily in the wavelength of light emitted by the particular active medium. The absorption of light by tissue varies according to wavelength. Thus the penetration of the incident laser beam and any consequent thermal or photochemical changes in tissue depends upon the wavelength of laser light produced and can be varied by the selection of a particular laser and according to how the energy is applied, i.e. whether continuously applied or in pulses of varying time duration.

As the applied light energy increases there is a primary thermal effect on the tissues. Initially, the tissue temperature rises and as energy is increased the tissue contracts, probably as a result of vaporization of water. With higher energies the cells are killed and ultimately the cellular material is vaporized leaving a tissue defect. This process, if continued, will bore a hole in the target tissue. When the surface layer of cells is injured there is also an area of milder cell damage underlying and adjacent to the target area. The extent of this zone of underlying cell damage depends on the type of laser used and on the variables discussed above; for example, the extent of the zone of underlying damage will be less below an area of CO_2 laser impact than below argon laser or Nd–YAG laser impact areas for the same given energy. Thus the essential difference between the three most commonly used lasers is the volume of the tissue that can be heated before the destruction of superficial cells occurs and this determines their clinical usefulness, i.e. the CO_2 laser can be used as a 'light scalpel' due to its localized effect with minimal damage to adjacent areas, whereas the Nd–YAG laser will heat a larger area and seal larger blood vessels.

The carbon dioxide (CO_2) laser

The CO_2 laser uses CO_2 molecules as the active medium and emits light with a wavelength of 10 600 nm in the invisible far infra-red portion of the electromagnetic spectrum. Laser energy of this wavelength is intensely absorbed by water; thus most of the incident energy will be absorbed in a thin surface layer of tissue. Since surface absorption is intense, scattering caused by refraction and reflection of the beam within the tissue will be negligible. Accordingly, the CO_2 laser produces heating and tissue vaporization at the point of impact so that successive thin layers of tissue are exposed to the laser and removed with minimal thermal injury below.

The focused beam can be used as a surgical cutter for making an incision without contact and in a relatively haemostatic manner. Characteristically small blood vessels (less than 0.1 mm diameter) will be coagulated by this cutting process but larger vessels are cut but not sealed and bleed freely, tending to interfere with subsequent tissue vaporization. Alternatively, if the beam is less focused a more diffuse heating effect is seen with less obvious tissue removal. By making the laser beam diameter wider the power density will fall and a slower, even more superficial vaporization over a larger surface area will result rather than precise deep cutting. This has been found to be a slow and inadequate method of tissue removal when applied to the prostate (Hall, 1982) via a suprapubic exposure. Unfortunately, the CO_2 laser wavelength is too long to allow fibre-optic transmission and rigid waveguides using a series of lenses and mirrors are used to conduct the energy where required. Together with the intense absorption of the energy by water this has made the CO_2 inappropriate for use in the watery urological environment even though high-power-output lasers are now available that might, in theory, deal more successfully with the prostate.

The argon laser

The argon laser produces plane, polarized light made up of a number of wavelengths lying between 437 nm and 529 nm with most power at 488 nm and 514 nm and is visible as a blue-green colour. The energy is selectively absorbed by pigmented lesions and by tissues with high blood content. The depth of penetration in tissues varies as a result of these factors, but as generally used is around 1.0 mm with greater haemostatic properties than the CO_2 laser but probably inadequate to deal with the vascular prostate. When active bleeding is present, the energy is rapidly absorbed by blood and the effective delivery of the laser beam to the underlying tissues is difficult. In practice it has been supplanted in general urological use by the Nd–YAG laser and will not be considered further.

Helium–neon laser

This low-power laser is now commonly used to provide a visual indication of the path of invisible wavelength laser beams such as the CO_2 and Nd–YAG and has no significant effect on tissues at the powers commonly available.

The dye laser

The dye laser is capable of generating a band of wavelengths depending on the physical characteristics of the particular dye used to produce the light. Wavelengths from the entire visible portion of the electromagnetic spectrum as well as wavelengths in the ultra-violet and infra-red portions are available. These devices permit the selection of wavelengths within the band and are to a limited degree 'tunable'. They are particularly used at present for the laser lithotripsy of urinary calculi and in the rapidly developing, but still largely experimental, field of photodynamic therapy (PDT) which in future may have a role in the treatment of prostate cancer (see below).

The neodymium–yttrium–aluminium–garnet (Nd–YAG) laser

The Nd–YAG laser uses a solid lasing medium of neodymium ions in an yttrium–aluminium–garnet crystal lattice. Nd–YAG lasers can generally emit a power of up to 100 W. The beam is invisible, but the point of impact is usually defined by the use of a visible red coaxial aiming beam produced by a low power helium–neon laser.

The Nd–YAG laser as most commonly used emits a wavelength of 1064 nm in the near infra-red region of the electromagnetic spectrum which is transmissible via a flexible quartz glass fibre by the process of total internal reflection. Light at this wavelength is not absorbed strongly by either water or body pigments (compared with the CO_2 and argon) but, because of the highly structured nature of body tissues, multiple reflections and refractions of the beam occur, resulting in a high degree of scattering. The net result is that a relatively large volume of tissue is affected by the laser energy about the point of beam impact.

As a result of its coagulative properties the Nd–YAG laser is particularly used in the endoscopic management of benign and malignant urological tumours and is the most commonly used urological laser.

Endoscopic Nd–YAG laser therapy

The Nd–YAG is the most readily usable laser for the urologist and lends itself to endoscopic use. The laser energy is conducted through fine flexible fibres which can be passed through the catheterizing channel of most urological instruments with minimal adaptation. Currently, laser treatment is directed largely at bladder tumours but several groups have developed endoscopic Nd–YAG laser therapies for benign and malignant disease of the prostate. These methods range from the simple endoscopic use of the fibre, through various beam-diverting devices, to the use of balloons in combination with laser light.

Endoscopic 'bare fibre' Nd–YAG laser therapy for prostate cancer

The relatively straightforward use of the bare fibre endoscopically has been advocated primarily for the treatment of localized prostate cancer. In the early 1980s Sander and Beisland described a novel technique (Sander *et al.*, 1982; Sander & Beisland, 1984) that combined a radical TURP to remove the bulk of tissue and 'de-bulk' the tumour, followed by endoscopic photocoagulation of the remaining prostatic capsule with the Nd-YAG laser in an attempt to sterilize any remaining cancer cells in the capsule.

Some comments on the background to this disease and the reasons for the development of this therapy are needed. The choice of a potentially curative treatment for early, apparently localized disease remains problematical. This is partly due to the difficulties inherent in trying to show a clear curative advantage for one modality over another in a condition with a prolonged and variable natural course. In addition, the condition is generally perceived as affecting a relatively elderly population of men and the morbidity of existing potentially curative treatment may be seen as excessive compared with benefits which remain unconvincing to many.

Both radiotherapy and radical surgery can both give rise to similar results in terms of survival in the best centres. Both radical surgery and radical radiotherapy have significant complications and side-effects. Radical surgery has been associated with an 85–90% chance of impotence (Walsh & Jewett, 1980) and a 10–15% incidence of incontinence (Smith & Kelly, 1984) although recent developments in methods of surgical removal of the gland, sparing the neurovascular bundles, have contributed to a reduction in the incidence of these serious complications (Walsh & Mostwin, 1984).

Radical radiotherapy commits the patient to a 6–8 week course of daily treatment, and even in the hands of the most experienced a significant complication rate of 10–12% has been reported (Ray & Bagshaw, 1975). Although long-term studies are not yet available seed implantation appears to be associated with a disease-free survival lower than that after radical surgery or radiotherapy; however, complications are similarly reduced (Nag, 1985).

Therefore, an alternative approach to curative therapy avoiding the morbidity of radical surgery or radiotherapy would be of great benefit. Ideally, such treatment would be endoscopic or 'minimally invasive' rather than requiring major open surgery. It would be applicable to prostatic tumour within any part of the gland, would have an acceptable incidence of side-effects, and particularly would have no adverse effects on potency or continence.

Sander and Beisland's novel endoscopic technique (Sander *et al.*, 1982; Sander & Beisland, 1984), combining a radical resection of the prostate to remove the bulk of tissue and 'de-bulk' the tumour with subsequent photocoagulation of the remaining prostatic capsule with the Nd–YAG laser to sterilize any remaining cancer cells in the capsule, looked like an interesting alternative approach as their initial results were encouraging in terms of disease-free survivals and there were no instances of impotence or incontinence (Beisland & Sander, 1986).

We have adapted this technique further in an attempt to extend the boundaries of endoscopic treatment for localized carcinoma of the prostate (McNicholas *et al.*, 1988a). In essence, following diagnosis of prostate cancer (usually at TURP) each man undergoes a second-look or 'extended' TURP done in planned and mapped segments. The purpose of this is firstly to 'de-bulk' the prostate gland under ultrasound control, aiming to leave a residual rim of prostatic capsule 6 mm or less in depth. In addition, this procedure allows further pathological staging.

Ten weeks later the patient undergoes Nd–YAG laser coagulation of his prostatic capsule. The energy is passed through a fine quartz glass fibre that is passed down the cystoscope or resectoscope and the whole surface of the capsular walls is irradiated using a power of 50 W and, when experience has increased, 60–70 W, slowly moving over the surface of the prostatic capsule in an attempt to evenly coagulate the whole area. The laser beam rests on any particular site for not more than 3–4 seconds at a time giving a depth of penetration of the laser energy of approximately 6 mm (Pensel *et al.*, 1981). At the start of that study we were guided by our experience of using the Nd–YAG laser in the bladder. However, it became clear that using 40 W for just 2 seconds in any one area (as in the bladder) seemed to have less of an effect than anticipated. This may have been partly because the healed prostatic cavity was quite white in appearance and may well have reflected a significant proportion of the laser energy. However, using those original parameters, the clinical impression was that not much heat was reaching the rectum, and this could be appreciated by the lack of heating of one's finger or of a thermocouple held against the anterior wall of the rectum and against the posterior lobe of the prostate. This was supported by the relatively minor changes seen endoscopically in the first few patients at 3 months following treatment.

As confidence increased we increased the power levels and spent much longer coagulating the prostatic capsule with the consequence that the total energy administered increased dramatically and reached levels of up to 50 000 J, higher than reported by the Oslo group (Sander & Beisland, 1986). Rectal temperature monitoring indicated temperatures reaching 52°C when lasering was stopped and the flow of irrigant increased. Transurethral access allowed adequate exposure of much of the prostatic capsule and of the bladder neck. However, for good access to the apical regions a suprapubic approach was also necessary (McNicholas *et al.*, 1988b).

After laser treatment patients were assessed at 1 month and were admitted for a full clinical, ultrasonic and endoscopic assessment at 3 months, 6 months and 1 year following treatment. Potency was assessed and serological tests for serum acid phosphatase (SAP), prostate specific antigen (PSA) and alkaline phosphatase were performed. They underwent endoscopy to monitor the healing of the prostatic capsule. Ultrasound-guided biopsies of any abnormal area and 'blind' transrectal biopsy of each lobe were taken in a determined effort to detect any cancer if present.

We have recently reviewed our experience of treating localized prostate cancer by endoscopic Nd–YAG laser coagulation (McNicholas & O'Donoghue, 1991). Twenty-two men have undergone a complete course of treatment ('extended' resection followed by laser coagulation of the prostatic cavity) with a mean follow-up of 38 months and all are at least 1 year post-treatment (range 25–50 months). The average age of the patients was 62.4 years, (range 39–75). These patients had, with one exception, either diffuse involvement of the gland (T0b or A2 disease) or had palpable and ultrasonic abnormalities putting them in a higher stage (T1–T2). It seems clear that those falling into the T0b (A2) group have a much more gloomy prognosis than the T0a (A1) and indeed than T1 disease (Sheldon *et al.*, 1980; Cantrell *et al.*, 1981; Beynon *et al.*, 1983) and merit consideration of more aggressive treatment rather than waiting for likely progression prior to instituting treatment. These patients form a population who might otherwise have been treated in the United Kingdom with external beam irradiation or, in many other countries, by radical prostatectomy.

In the early stages of follow-up two patients had positive biopsies. In both cases clinical, ultrasonic and endoscopic evidence suggested that an excess of tissue had been left. They have both undergone further de-bulking TURP and second laser treatments with negative biopsies subsequently. Two patients have clinical and pathological evidence of remaining apical disease and in retrospect were understaged despite our best efforts and would not have been suitable for any local therapy given with curative intent. The other patients have negative biopsies.

We have measured PSA levels in 13 patients prior to treatment and 22 have had PSA levels measured following laser treatment up until June 1990. In 14, values measured at least 6 months after treatment have dropped into the same range as that following successful total prostatectomy for localized disease ($<0.5\,\mu g/l$, Hybritech, San Diego, California). Two (9%) are above $4\,\mu g/l$, the upper limit of normal and these are the two clear failures on clinical and pathological grounds. Overall, 16 men (72%) have PSA levels within the range of PSA values that are 'undetectable' by the two available assays.

There appears to be unanimity in the literature that successful removal of all prostatic epithelial tissue, whether in the pelvis or elsewhere, should be marked by a reduction of PSA levels below the previously quoted 'normal' range and into an 'undetectable' range (Hudson *et al.*, 1989). This range is quoted by Hybritech as $<0.5\,\mu g/l$. The significance of these results is that it strongly implies the absence of any significant prostatic acinar epithelial cells within the residual post-laser prostate.

To put these PSA levels after endoscopic laser therapy into context it is important to realize that these levels are those one would expect after a successful (i.e. complete) radical prostatectomy for truly localized, intraglandular disease. Such low levels are not often achieved by the other potentially curative options. Hudson *et al.* (1989) describe how infrequently the PSA values of their patients went into 'undetectable levels' after radiotherapy that was apparently or intended to be curative. Only three of 18 patients (17%) had post-irradiation PSA values of less than 0.6 ng/ml (or 0.6 μg/l) while in 39% PSA remained between 4 and 10 μg/l with 22% (four of 18) of values being greater than 10 μg/l. Stamey *et al.* (1987) describe 108 patients receiving radiotherapy at Stanford and found that in only 13% did PSA values fall into the undetectable range and in only 35% did the PSA return to the normal reference range.

Characteristically, the whole gland is much shrunken, both in total length and in its A–P diameter. The volume changes during the stages of the treatment and during follow-up reveal that the average volume of the gland at diagnosis was 24.4 cm^3 (17–38 cm^3) and after the second-look or extended TURP 14 cm^3 (9.4–22.3 cm^3), falling at 3 months after laser treatment to 7.5 cm^3 (2.3–19.5 cm^3). Overall, therefore, we recorded a 70% reduction in the volume of the prostate gland.

An endoscopic 'extensive' or 'radical' TURP intending to remove all prostatic tissue, both adenoma and true prostatic gland tissue, leaving only the prostatic capsule, is fraught with technical problems: most importantly the difficulties in truly removing all the tissue that is intended for removal, and secondly the fact that severe haemorrhage from pericapsular vessels may be encountered. This method overcomes these problems by allowing an extensive ultrasound-guided resection that remains generally within the bounds of the prostate but allows complete coagulation of the residual prostatic 'rim' by means of the laser. Tissues beyond the prostate, including the pelvic autonomic nerves, may be protected by the 'heat sink' effect of the pericapsular and more distant vessels, whereas diathermy may be relatively concentrated on these vascular channels, leading to the potential for concentration of current and resultant thermal injury. The rectum is also protected by the presence of the Denonvilliers fascia (and the pelvic plexus nerves responsible for potency may be protected by the vasa nervorum and the veins of Santorini's plexus).

The possibility that TURP and in particular a second-look, radical or extended TURP as described could have an adverse influence on the prognosis of prostate cancer has to be considered. It is conceivable that, particularly as one reaches the outer limits of the prostate, and tends to impinge on the relatively large-bore low-pressure venous sinuses, then viable tumour cell material could be liberated, and might find its way into these vessels and thence disseminate. Dissemination of viable prostatic tumour cells after TURP has been reported by Cole *et al.* (1961) who found cancer cells in the inferior vena cava following TURP, and by Miedena & Redman (1981) who found pulmonary emboli of prostatic cancer, believed to be a direct result of TURP.

There is a significant literature in which the possible relationship between the method of achieving histological confirmation of the diagnosis and the eventual outcome have been considered. In 1980 McGowan noted an increased recurrence rate in patients treated with radiation therapy for early stages B and C prostatic cancers when diagnosis had been done by transurethral resection, rather than by needle biopsy. Hanks *et al.* (1983) similarly revealed an adverse effect of TURP in patients with T3 and T4 cancers. However, there was a clear increase in the number of poorly differentiated cancers in the TURP group compared with the needle biopsy group. Schwemmer *et al.* (1986), in their study using a multivariate analysis model incorporating tumour grade and stage, found TURP to be without effect on survival rates or on the interval to distant or local recurrence after adjustments had been made for the effects of stage and grade. Paulson & Cox (1987) and Meacham *et al.* (1989) looked at 145 patients and 379 patients respectively. They found no difference in time to evidence of failure and concluded TURP does not enhance the appearance of metastatic disease.

The balance of opinion would seem to favour there being no significant deleterious effect from TURP *per se* but rather that those requiring TURP have rather extensive or more biologically threatening disease. These patients would be more likely to have symptoms of outflow obstruction and this may account for why they underwent TURP more frequently than needle biopsy. Of course tumour is also more likely to be already present in lymph nodes and more distantly than in smaller-volume prostatic cancers.

It is too early to make any suggestion as to the overall efficacy of this technique. In addition, the method has been altered, there being a steady increase in total energy given as experience has increased, and as we became aware that the earliest patients had been relatively under-treated. These energy totals are much higher than those described by H.O. Beisland (pers. comm., 1988) but we consider them essential to reliably achieve a sufficiently deep effect over the whole surface area of the prostatic cavity.

The extent of resection increased in a similar fashion, with increasing familiarity with the ultrasound guidance and with subsequent evidence that, again, the earliest patients had been inadequately resected.

The two cases of clear treatment failures had residual tumour in their apical region. Apical tissue remains a challenge to this method of treatment, especially if the prostatic apical tissue is seen to extend significantly below the level of the verumontanum. This part of the prostate is often the site of tumour (Byar & Mostofi, 1972). Complete apical resection may be difficult to achieve by the transurethral route without compromising the external sphincter. Attention is currently being directed to more radical methods of performing the final resection of apical tissue, both from below and from the suprapubic track, which has the advantage of allowing resection to proceed in a direction away from the sphincter mechanism rather than always towards it as in transurethral resection (McNicholas *et al.*, 1988b; Sanchez de Badajoz & Perez-Castro, 1991). Resection can be guided by the ultrasound image on which the sphincter and resectoscope can both be clearly identified.

Although any treatment for carcinoma of the prostate must be judged over a prolonged period of follow-up, the method in its present state of development has resulted in 88% of the treated patients having no evidence of disease despite careful and repeated biopsy and EUA (examination under anaesthetic). The treatment described can be repeated, has not affected continence and has, in our experience, a low incidence of impotence.

Endoscopic Nd–YAG laser therapy for benign adenomatous enlargement

Bare fibre Simply pointing the Nd–YAG laser fibre towards the benign prostatic adenoma and expecting to see an effect seemed a bit too simple and straightforward to be significantly effective at overcoming prostatic obstruction. Certainly we were not impressed by the immediate effects when we experimented this way. Hall (1982) found the Nd–YAG laser used on the prostate at 50 W to be relatively ineffective as a tissue remover and was unable to prevent bleeding or to achieve satisfactory haemostasis. Our experiments suggested that the immediate tissue-removing power of the Nd–YAG was less under fluid than in air, in addition to which, it was suspected that even if a significant volume of necrosis was produced it would slough over a period of days or weeks. This possibility was not encouraging as the chronic problems of sloughing following cryotherapy of the prostate had largely accounted for that process not achieving widespread popularity. However, two recent developments which may have improved the 'geometry' of Nd–YAG laser energy application to the prostate suggest that these fears may have been exaggerated.

Fibre beam deflector devices Costello *et al.* (1991) have recently presented their preliminary findings in a study of endoscopic Nd–YAG lasering where the beam passing from the distal end of the fibre is deflected off a miniature gold-plated alloy reflector 'mirror' close to the end of the fibre so that it strikes the target adenoma almost perpendicularly. This may improve the transmission of the energy to the tissues, compared with the bare fibre method where the beam usually strikes the target surface obliquely due to the orientation of the endoscope and fibre. They showed a surprising degree of immediate tissue removal and encouraging but very early results in which symptoms improved even though there was little change in the flow rates. Though more tissue slough came away subsequently it did not appear to be a problem for their patients. This method has the advantage of being relatively simple and well within the capabilities of most urologists with access to an Nd–YAG laser.

Balloon devices The coagulation effect of the Nd–YAG laser beam in prostatic tissue can be increased by ensuring that the beam strikes the target as close to the perpendicular as possible. The efficiency of energy transfer into the prostate can be increased further by firing the laser beam from a fixed central point through a transparent balloon. A balloon distended within the prostatic fossa seems to act in a manner that flattens out the prostatic urethral lining and probably improves the 'geometry' of Nd–YAG laser energy application to the prostate and compresses the tissue, reducing its vascularity, i.e. the beam strikes a constant-sized portion of the prostate surface which is relatively flat and relatively ischaemic. The Intra-Sonix 'TULIP' (transurethral laser-induced prostatectomy; Burlington, Massachusetts) device has been designed to provide right-angled Nd–YAG laser beam delivery through a 36–48 F balloon pressurized to 2 atmospheres (202 kPa) to take advantage of these features. In addition, the laser treatment is directed by endoscopic transurethral ultrasound emitted and received by miniature transducers incorporated within the 20 F transurethral probe and situated so that the beam is always at the centre of the ultrasound image. Once the operator is familiar with the ultrasonic features of the bladder neck and apex of the prostate s/he can pull the device through the gland repeatedly, causing a number of linear areas of laser coagulation. Animal studies have been impressive (Assimos *et al.*, 1991) but results derived from the canine prostate do tend to flatter and the 'proof of the pudding' is, can these effects be reproduced in man?

The laser part of the procedure may be completed in a few minutes and the patient can be discharged immediately though usually with a catheter for a short period. Exactly how long the catheter is required is unclear and varies between the centres evaluating the 'TULIP'. Only very early follow-up results are available (Roth *et al.*, 1991) but there does appear to be an improvement in symptom scores and a rather less marked increase in flow rates. The tissue sloughing that does occur has not been a significant problem for the patients treated so far.

There are other balloon devices in development including a device that uses the Nd–YAG laser beam to heat fluid in the balloon which then heats the prostate. This is not yet clinically available and has been hampered by quality control problems with the balloon, leading to unexpected rupture (Watson G.M., pers. comm., 1991).

Interstitial laser coagulation for benign and malignant disease of the prostate

As an alternative to the endoscopic use of the Nd–YAG laser our recent research efforts have focused on the feasibility of using implanted fibres to conduct relatively low-power Nd–YAG laser light to cause the localized coagulative necrosis of prostatic tissue.

Malignant prostatic disease

McNeal's work (McNeal *et al.*, 1986) has suggested that tumours start small and well differentiated. As they grow they lose differentiation and acquire the capacity for metastases, probably expressed largely in those above 1 ml in volume. Thus it appears that carcinoma of the prostate does indeed follow a predictable course. The clinically undetected 'latent cancers' reported from the post-mortem series are not, therefore, a separate disease entity but are in most cases recent developments (as a manifestation of the sharply rising age-specific incidence curve), and are too small to be detectable or to have achieved metastatic potential. It follows that the presence of prostatic cancer in the younger man does put him at risk of disease progression, even if the extent of the tumour is apparently very small, purely by virtue of his longer time at risk.

Adami *et al.* (1986) have also suggested that clinically diagnosed carcinoma of the prostate does not behave in 'benign fashion' even at an advanced age and does in fact significantly affect survival whenever diagnosed.

The challenge to the clinician is whether s/he can pick out those at particularly high risk of significant tumour development. An encouraging finding of McNeal's report (McNeal *et al.*, 1986) is that the features to which metastatic potential was related, i.e. volume, depth and extent of capsular invasion and seminal vesicle involvement, are all increasingly measurable or detectable with ultrasound and particularly transrectal ultrasound (TRUS).

TRUS increasingly allows the detection of small, potentially malignant areas within the prostate gland which can be precisely biopsied under ultrasound control for an accurate tissue diagnosis and histological grading (Lee *et al.*, 1985). This opens up the possibility of increased accuracy of prognosis and may allow direction of curative therapy to younger men or to those with small-volume disease who can more reliably be expected not to have already developed metastatic spread.

As stated before, an alternative approach to curative therapy, avoiding the morbidity of radical surgery or radiotherapy and yet capable of dealing effectively with low-volume disease, would be of great interest, particularly if a tumoricidal stimulus could be administered through fine needles. Of especial interest would be if the treatment and its effects could be monitored ultrasonically and the patient then remain under surveillance and receive repeat treatments if new lesions developed. It would have to be applicable to prostatic tumour within any part of the gland. Also, it would have to have an acceptable incidence of side-effects, and particularly have no adverse effects on potency or continence if it is to be offered to younger men than those usually met in our clinics.

Nd–YAG laser light was suggested for the purpose of creating focal areas of tissue coagulation within a solid organ (Bown, 1983). We are currently investigating whether sources of laser light can be placed via fine fibre-optic fibres within the prostate gland to cause precise, controlled necrosis of a size that might be useful for the treatment of small prostatic cancers.

Prostatic heating can be performed by a variety of methods such as microwave, radiofrequency, ultrasound and whole body. The problem with these alternatives is largely one of accuracy of application, in other words, getting the energy to the tumour and delivering adequate energy to cause the required temperatures for long enough to result in cell death. The advantage of the interstitial laser technique described below is that the energy is easily placed into the tissue, the fibre being of a small and relatively non-traumatic size.

Preliminary clinical studies (Steger *et al.*, 1989) have shown the feasibility of such a technique in clinical trials of Nd–YAG laser coagulation of tumours of the pancreas and liver. It is crucial that truly localized coagulation is created and for that to be achieved the positioning of fibres must be extremely accurate. These clinical studies and our own experimental studies (McNicholas *et al.*, 1988c; 1991) of the same technique used on the prostate have shown that the needles used for fibre implantation, the fibres used and the effect caused and the healed lesions can show up on ultrasound, allowing accurate positioning and offering the possibility of watching the process from beginning to end on an ultrasound screen and so ensuring precise obliteration of the suspicious area.

During the experiments one or more 150–400 μm diameter fibres were implanted within the substance of the elderly male beagle prostate. Nd–YAG laser energy could be transmitted through the fibre(s) using longer exposures (200 s–1500 s) and lower powers than used in routine endoscopic laser therapy. Well-defined areas of coagulative necrosis could be created without extensive tissue charring or damage to the fibre. For an energy dose of 1000 J a lesion approximately 1 cm in diameter resulted at 4 days, i.e. lesion size approximated to that of truly early, localized prostate cancers. Treatments were well tolerated. At 6 weeks following treatment, healing was by fibrosis surrounding an area of cystic degeneration. Performing experiments with multiple fibres implanted produced larger-volume lesions relevant to more extensive cancer or for the coagulation of benign adenomatous hyperplasia causing outflow symptoms.

However, there is an enormous difference between the soft, glandular canine prostate and the human gland with its glandular, muscular and stromal elements which is more resistant to heating and other 'minimally invasive' therapies. It is not wise to extrapolate from canine results to the human and further clinical experiments are under way to determine the response of the human prostate to interstitial laser heating in clinical studies as well as to answer the question of whether we could see (ultrasonically) the needles and fibres, and, most fundamentally, whether the ILC heating effect itself could be seen.

We performed temperature measurement studies to determine the response of the human prostate to an interstitial thermal effect, to measure the spread of heat through the gland and to find out if therapeutically useful temperatures could be achieved despite the known high blood flow in the gland.

Patients undergoing pelvic lymph node dissection and radical prostatectomy in our unit and who gave fully informed consent underwent insertion of a laser fibre and needle microthermocouples into the surgically exposed prostate gland whilst surgery was halted awaiting the results of frozen section examination of the pelvic lymph nodes.

Each thermocouple and laser fibre was placed into the prostate under direct vision with additional TRUS imaging so that their positions relative to one another could be assessed and measured clinically and by ultrasound. The appearances of the TRUS images were recorded on videotape. A standard treatment of 1000 J was given whilst measuring temperatures and observing ultrasound changes.

We found that a well-localized area of heated tissue developed which had characteristic TRUS appearances. Within seconds of the start of treatment with the laser a focus of 'bright', hyperechoic tissue developed and expanded gradually outward from the tip of the laser fibre. Once laser heating stopped then the hyperechoic zone stopped growing and began to shrink. Measurements of the lateral extent of the hyperechoic zone suggest dimensions greater than 1.5 cm in diameter.

The temperature distribution data during ILC showed a relatively regular lateral spread of thermal effect. The thermal effect spread out to approximately 2 cm from the point source where recorded temperatures approached normal, suggesting that the lateral extent of a necrosing effect would approach 2 cm, at which point adjacent tissues would be relatively unaffected, i.e. the thermal injury is quite localized and also the zone of significantly raised temperature appears to approximate to the dimensions of the ultrasound visible zone of hyperechogenicity.

Benign prostatic disease

It is perhaps not surprising that interstitial laser coagulation has been considered for the destruction of benign adenomatous hyperplasia of the prostate. Because of the importance of benign prostatic hypertrophy the study was extended to determine whether larger volumes of tissue (corresponding to the enlarged benign adenoma) could also be destroyed in the same manner. The fundamental approach of this project is to use the same basic interstitial method, that is, to cause localized coagulation of prostatic tissue in a precise, controlled manner over a relatively short period of time, in a way that can be observed during the coagulative process and with results that can be seen and assessed on follow-up.

For coagulation of a significant portion of the benign prostatic adenoma the effect must be placed within the main mass of the endoscopic lateral lobe adenoma (or McNeal's transition zone tissue) but sufficiently far away from the sphincter areas and the pelvic plexus nerves controlling potency. It would appear that the lateral lobe of the prostate should be the prime target (and this implies excluding patients with middle lobe prostatic enlargement since this group have not done well with any of the 'non-surgical' methods of prostatic therapy available).

This effect seen in the laboratory models exceeds that shown by the microwave techniques previously described at scientific meetings and is similar to the most effective microwave machine we have seen so far. It has the advantage of involving only one treatment, being easily combined with endoscopic review and using relatively cheap equipment (TRUS, Nd–YAG laser) often already available to the urologist.

Clinical application is in its early stages in our unit with encouraging preliminary results and no significant complications. It is our impression that this method will be most effective in the symptomatic and yet not severely obstructed man with a relatively modest benign prostatic enlargement who may experience deterioration temporarily due to prostatic oedema before he notes improvement. Obviously these caveats apply to most, if not all, of the currently available 'non-surgical' therapeutic options.

Photodynamic therapy (PDT)

PDT involves the use of lasers to produce pure light wavelengths chosen to cause activation of previously administered photosensitizing agents to cause cell injury by a non-thermal mechanism. Ideally, the photosensitizing drug is taken up or retained to a greater degree by malignant tissue than by normal tissue. Several agents have this potential but haematoporphyrin, a non-metallic porphyrin derived from haemoglobin, has been the most completely investigated.

Early investigators found that intravenous haematoporphyrin tended to localize in malignant tissues as could be noted from the fact that tumour cells would fluoresce as a red colour when exposed to near ultra-violet light (± 405 nm). 'Haematoporphyrin derivative' (HpD) has a greater affinity for malignant tissue than haematoporphyrin. HpD was not only a tumour localization agent, but also an active photosensitizing agent. Cytotoxicity would occur in cells that had taken up HpD if they were exposed to wavelengths of light corresponding to the peaks of the absorption spectrum of HpD.

The precise mechanism by which the tumour cells are killed is unclear but probably involves the liberation of oxygen radicals and toxic effects on small blood vessels (Star *et al.*, 1986). Any source of light of the appropriate wavelength and power output may be used for PDT. Red light (630 nm) would be attractive for lesions situated within the prostate because it penetrates the tissue more deeply. Obviously when the depth of the lesion is less, e.g. superficial carcinoma *in situ* of the bladder, a wavelength with a lower penetration such as blue light (400 nm) which corresponds to the highest absorption band of HpD or blue-green (500 nm) would be preferred.

The timing of light delivery after HpD administration has varied in the clinical studies reported dealing with the bladder. Most investigators treat within 48 to 72 hours after administration of an intravenous dose of HpD.

Because the skin absorbs a quantity of HpD sufficient to produce a marked photosensitivity, i.e. sunburn, every patient must be carefully and repeatedly warned to avoid exposure to sunlight and to cover exposed parts of the body for up to 4 weeks. Thus the United Kingdom may be one of the most appropriate sites in the world for this treatment modality! More recently other photosensitizing agents such as thiocyanates have been evaluated in the search for a greater differential absorption by tumour from normal cells with less toxicity (Bown *et al.*, 1986).

The techniques of accurate needle (and fibre) insertion throughout the prostate are established — for radioactive seed implantation, for example. It would appear logical to extend interstitial methods further and attempt to illuminate the entire prostate following administration of a photosensitizer. This experimental project is very much at the laboratory stage as yet but has been stimulated by the increasing awareness of the 'transparency' of the prostate to certain wavelengths (Pantelides *et al.*, 1990).

Conclusion

The use of laser energy for the treatment of prostatic problems has undergone an enormous recent revival with the refinement of methods to make the laser processes more predictable and controllable. The possibilities look encouraging. However, a great deal more experience of each variant is required before it will be clear whether these laser methods have a role to play in prostatic disease and which of them are most appropriate to benign or malignant pathology.

References

Adami H.O., Norlen B.J., Malker B. & Meirik O. (1986) Long term survival in prostatic carcinoma with special reference to age as a prognostic factor. *Scand. J. Urol. Nephrol.*, **20**, 107–12.

Assimos D.G., McCullough D.L., Woodruff R.D., Harrison L.H., Hart L.J. & Li W.J. (1991) Canine transurethral laser induced prostatectomy. *J. Endourol.*, **5**, 145–9.

Beisland H.O. & Sander S. (1986) First clinical experiences on neodymium–YAG laser irradiation of localised prostatic carcinoma. *Scand. J. Urol. Nephrol.*, **20**, 113–17.

Beynon L.L., Busuttil A., Newsam J.E. & Chisholm G.D. (1983) Incidental carcinoma of the prostate: selection for deferred treatment. *Br. J. Urol.*, **55**, 733–6.

Bown S.G. (1983) Phototherapy of tumours. *World J. Surg.*, **7**, 700–9.

Bown S.G., Trelau C.J., Coleridge-Smith P.D., Akdemir D. & Wieman T.J. (1986) Photodynamic therapy with porphyrin and pthallocyanine sensitisation: quantitative studies in normal rat liver. *Br. J. Cancer*, **54**, 43–52.

Byar D.P. & Mostofi F.K. (1972) Carcinoma of the prostate: prognostic evaluation of certain pathologic features in 208 radical prostatectomies. *Cancer*, **30**, 5–13.

Cantrell B.B., DeKlerk D.P., Eggleston J.C., Boitnott J.K. & Walsh P.C. (1981) Pathological factors that influence prognosis in stage A prostatic cancer: the influence of extent versus grade. *J. Urol.*, **125**, 516–20.

Cole W.H., McDonald G.O., Roberts S.S. & Southwick H.W. (1961) *Dissemination of Cancer: Prevention and Therapy*, p. 143. Appleton–Century–Crofts, New York.

Costello A.J., Johnson D.E., Bolton D.M. & Bowsher W.G. (1991) Nd–YAG laser ablation of the prostate as a treatment for benign prostatic hypertrophy. Presentation to: British Association of Urological Surgeons Annual Meeting, Glasgow, 28 June 1991 (Abstract 156).

Hall R.R. (1982) Report to the standing committee on urological instruments: Lasers in urology. *Br. J. Urol.*, **54**, 421–6.

Hanks G.E., Leibel S. & Kramer S. (1983) Dissemination of cancer by transurethral resection of locally advanced prostate cancer. *J. Urol.*, **129**, 309–11.

Hudson M.A., Bahnson R.B. & Catalona W.J. (1989) Clinical use of prostate specific antigen in patients with prostate cancer. *J. Urol.*, **142**, 1011–17.

Lee F., Gray J.M., McLeary R.D., Meadows T.R., Kumasaka G.H., Borlaza G.S., Straub W.H., Lee F., Solomon M.H., McHugh T.A. & Wolf R.M. (1985) Transrectal ultrasound in the diagnosis of prostate cancer: location, echogenicity, histopathology and staging. *The Prostate*, **7**, 117–29.

McGowan D.G. (1980) The adverse influence of prior TUR in prognosis of carcinoma of the prostate treated by radiotherapy. *Int. J. Radiat. Oncol. Biol. Phys.*, **6**, 1121–4.

McNeal J.E., Kindrachuk R.A., Freiha F.S., Bostwick D.G., Redwine E.A. & Stamey T.A. (1986) Patterns of progression in prostate cancer. *Lancet*, **i**, 60–3.

McNicholas T.A. & O'Donoghue E.P.N. (1991) Endoscopic YAG laser coagulation for early prostate cancer. Proceedings of the International Society for Optical Engineering. SPIE's *Biomedical Optics*, Vol. 1421, *Lasers in Urology, Laparoscopy and General Surgery*. SPIE Optical Engineering Press, Bellingham, WA, USA (in press).

McNicholas T.A., Steger A.C., Charig C. & Bown S.G. (1988a) Interstitial Yag laser coagulation of the prostate. *Lasers Med. Sci. Abstracts Issue,* Abstract 446.

McNicholas T.A., Ramsay J.W.A., Carter S.St.C. & Miller R.A. (1988b) Suprapubic endoscopy: a percutaneous approach. *Br. J. Urol.,* **61**, 221–3.

McNicholas T.A., Carter S.St.C., Wickham J.E.A. & O'Donoghue E.P.N. (1988c) YAG laser treatment of early carcinoma of the prostate. *Br. J. Urol.,* **61**, 239–43.

McNicholas T.A., Steger A.C, Pope A., Bown S.G. & O'Donoghue N. (1991) Interstitial laser coagulation of the prostate: experimental studies. Proceedings of the International Society for Optical Engineering. SPIE's *Biomedical Optics,* Vol. 1421, *Lasers in Urology, Laparoscopy and General Surgery.* SPIE Optical Engineering Press, Bellingham, WA, USA.

Meacham R.B., Scardino P.T., Hoffman G.S., Easley J.D., Wilbanks J.H. & Carlton C.E. (1989) The risk of distant metastases after transurethral resection of the prostate versus needle biopsy in patients with localised prostate cancer. *J. Urol.,* **142**, 320–5.

Miedena E.B. & Redman J.F. (1981) Microscopic pulmonary embolization by adenocarcinoma of the prostate. *Urology,* **18**, 399–401.

Nag S. (1985) Radioactive I 125 implantation for carcinoma of the prostate. *The Prostate,* **6**, 293–301.

Pantelides M., Whiteburst C., Moore J.V., King T.A. & Blacklock N.J. (1990) Photodynamic therapy for localised prostate cancer: light penetration in the human prostate gland. *J. Urol.,* **143**, 398–401.

Paulson D.F. & Cox E.B. (1987) Does transurethral resection of the prostate promote metastatic disease? *J. Urol.,* **138**, 90–1.

Pensel J., Hofstetter A., Keiditsch E. & Rothenberger K. (1981) Temporal and spatial temperature profile of the bladder serosa in intravesical neodymium YAG laser irradiation. *Eur. Urol.,* **7**, 298–303.

Ray G.R. & Bagshaw M.A. (1975) The role of radiation therapy in the definitive treatment of adenocarcinoma of the prostate. *Ann. Rev. Med.,* **26**, 567–88.

Roos N.P., Wennberg J.E., Malenka D.J., Fisher E.S., McPherson K., Andersen T.F., Cohen M.M. & Ramsey E. (1989) Mortality and reoperation after open and transurethral resection of the prostate for benign prostatic hyperplasia. *New Engl. J. Med.* **320**, 1120–4.

Roth R.A., Babayan R. & Aretz T. (1991) TULIP — transurethral ultrasound guided laser induced prostatecomy. Presentation to American Urological Association, Toronto, 5 June 1991. *J. Urol.,* **145**, 390A (Abstract 712).

Sanchez de Badajoz E. & Perez-Castro E. (1991) Suprapubic resection of the prostate. *J. Endourol.,* **5**, 157–9.

Sander S. & Beisland H.O. (1984) Laser in the treatment of localised prostatic carcinoma. *J. Urol.,* **132**, 280–1.

Sander S., Beisland H.O. & Fossberg E. (1982) Neodymium YAG laser in the treatment of prostatic cancer. *Urol. Res.,* **10**, 85–6.

Schwemmer B., Ulm K., Rotter M., Braen J. & Schultz W. (1986) Does transurethral resection of prostatic carcinoma promote tumour spread? *Urol. Int.,* **41**, 284–8.

Sheldon C.A., Williams R.D. & Fraley E.E. (1980) Incidental carcinoma of the prostate: a review of the literature and critical reappraisal of classification. *J. Urol.,* **124**, 626–31.

Smith J.M. & Kelly D.G. (1984) Radical prostatectomy in the management of localised carcinoma of the prostate. *Br. J. Urol.,* **56**, 690–3.

Stamey T.A., Yang N., Hay A.R., McNeal J.E., Freiha F.S. & Redwine E.

(1987) Prostate specific antigen as a serum marker for adenocarcinoma of the prostate. *New Engl. J. Med.*, **317**, 909–16.

Star W.M., Marijnissen H.P.A., van der Berg-Blok A.E., Versteeg J.A.C., Franken K.A.P. & Reinhold H.S. (1986) Destruction of rat mammary tumour and normal tissue microcirculation by haematoporphyrin derivative photoradiation observed *in vivo* in sandwich observation chambers. *Cancer Research*, **46**, 2532–40.

Steger A.C., Lees W.R., Walmsley K. & Bown S.G. (1989) Interstitial laser hyperthermia: a new approach to local destruction of tumours. *Br. Med. J.*, **299**, 362–5.

Walsh P.C. & Jewett H.J. (1980) Radical surgery for prostatic cancer. *Cancer*, **45**, 1906–11.

Walsh P.C. & Mostwin J.L. (1984) Radical prostatectomy and cystoprostatectomy with preservation of potency: results using a new nerve sparing technique. *Br. J. Urol.*, **56**, 694–7.

Index